# Uncovered

## Stories from the Skin-Difference Community

An Anthology

# Uncovered

## Stories from the Skin-Difference Community
### An Anthology

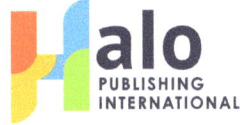

Copyright © 2025 Hanna Prangner (Compiler and Manager). All rights reserved.

No part of this publication may be reproduced, stored in a retrieval system or transmitted in any form or by any means, electronic, mechanical, photocopying, recording or otherwise, without prior permission of Halo Publishing International.

The views and opinions expressed in this book are those of the author and do not necessarily reflect the official policy or position of Halo Publishing International. Any content provided by our authors are of their opinion and are not intended to malign any religion, ethnic group, club, organization, company, individual or anyone or anything.

No generative artificial intelligence (AI) was used in the writing of this work. The author expressly prohibits any entity from using this publication to train AI technologies to generate text, including, without limitation, technologies capable of generating works in the same style or genre as this publication.

For permission requests, write to the publisher, addressed "Attention: Permissions Coordinator," at the address below.

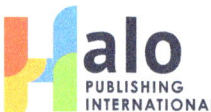

Halo Publishing International
7550 W IH-10 #800, PMB 2069,
San Antonio, TX 78229

First Edition, May 2025
ISBN: 978-1-63765-776-8
Library of Congress Control Number: 2025908367

Halo Publishing International is a self-publishing company that publishes adult fiction and non-fiction, children's literature, self-help, spiritual, and faith-based books. Do you have a book idea you would like us to consider publishing? Please visit www.halopublishing.com for more information.

# CONTENTS

| | |
|---|---|
| **AUTHORS** | 11 |
| **MY PORT-WINE STORY**<br>Ana Lankford | 13 |
| **DEATH KNOCKED ON MY DOOR ELEVEN TIMES**<br>Batool Kaushal | 23 |
| **AMAZING AMELIA**<br>Crystal Gordon | 35 |
| **A SHORT STORY ABOUT CONFIDENCE**<br>Dana Marie Rückert | 47 |
| **THE JOURNEY**<br>Hanna Prangner | 57 |
| **THE DAY I LEARNED MY NAME**<br>J. Brian | 65 |

## BIRTHMARKED BADASS ... 73
Jessica Weckherlin

## STICKS AND STONES ... 89
Kirsty Heather Ferguson

## HOW I STOPPED LETTING MY BIRTHMARK DEFINE ME ... 97
Lorena Bryant Hixson

## MY STORY: BEYOND THE STARES ... 107
Matthias De Potter

## MY STORY, MY JOURNEY ... 115
Omaima Aladwani

## MY STORY, MY PAIN, AND MY GLORY ... 119
Penny Pellens

## HOW I FOUND YOU GUYS ... 129
Dr. Scott Cupples

## MY STORY: FROM PATIENT TO HELPER ... 139
Sharon James

## MY SIXTH SENSE: MY PORT-WINE STAIN ... 145
Simran Kaur Dhatt

**SMILE AND SAY CHEESE!** 157
Tiffany Kerchner

**ABOUT THE AUTHORS** 165

# AUTHORS

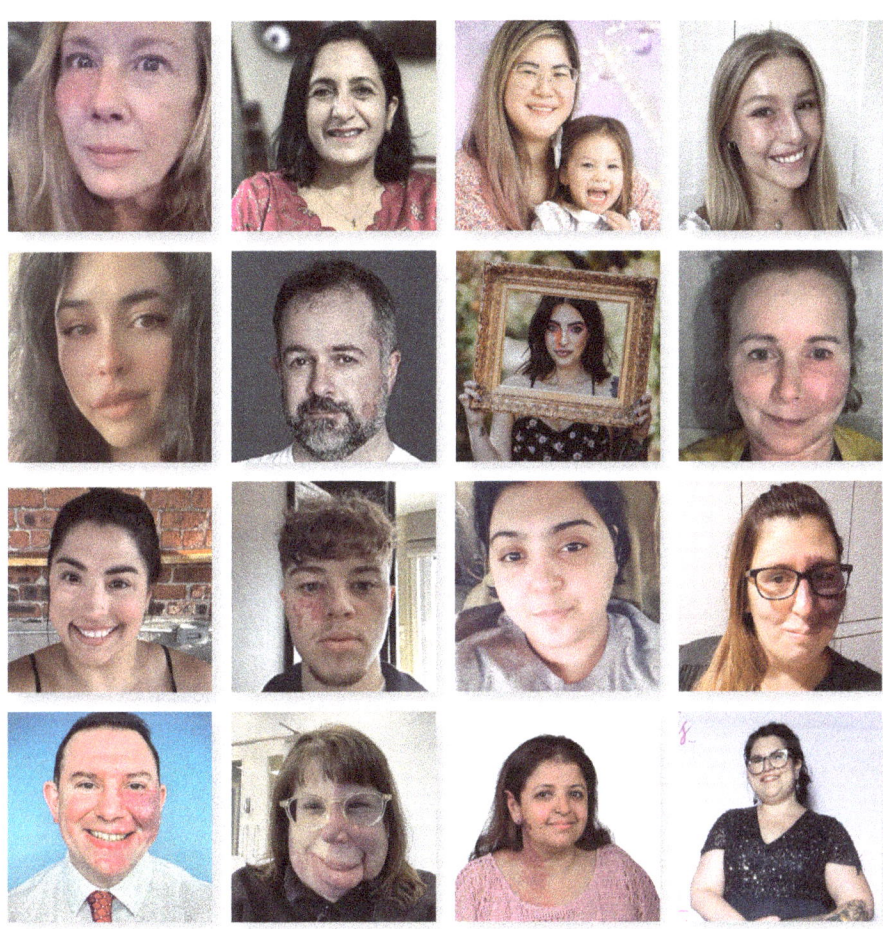

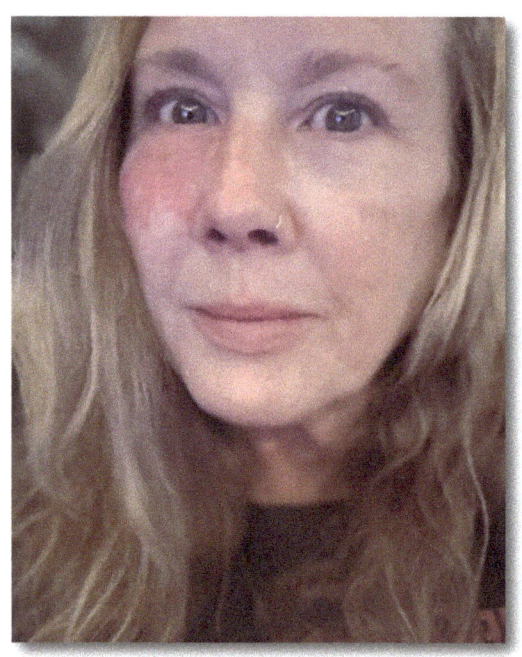

"I have learned to embrace the inherent beauty in being different. The world is full of imperfections, and those imperfections are what bring beauty to the world."

# MY PORT-WINE STORY
## Ana Lankford

I was born in 1967, on a sunny June day in Oklahoma City. My mom jokes to this day about my always being in a rush, and my birth was the start, as I was almost born in the street in front of the hospital! My birthmark is on my left cheek and covers about one-fourth of my cheek. My PWS does go into my eye and thus my brain. I have not been given a formal Sturge-Weber diagnosis; however, my doctor suspects it is present due to the higher pressure in my eye and the cluster headaches I have experienced. A formal diagnosis has not been important to me, as I do not have seizures and other symptoms.

Growing up, I was fairly protected. I do recall times in grade school when I was called Cherry Kool-Aid Face, but overall my elementary years were fairly calm. It was when I entered middle school that things really began to change, and I fully realized how different I actually was. Prior to middle school, I had had some negative interactions with the public.

One in particular that still stands out to me is being in line at the grocery store with my mom. I was around six or seven years old at the time. The woman in line ahead of us kept staring at me, and my mom noticed. She smiled at the lady and said, "Isn't my daughter beautiful?"

The woman looked my mom in the eye and said, "No, she is not; she has been marked by Satan as his."

My mother is the kindest, gentlest human you can meet, but in that moment, I saw the protective tiger she was and is. I believe that was the moment I also knew not everyone was kind and something was truly different about me.

High school is when it became really hard for me. I can remember praying every night for God to take my birthmark off my face and put it anywhere else—my neck, shoulder, arm, leg—just anywhere but my face. When I looked in the mirror, I hated what I saw. Daily in school, my only goal was to be invisible and just make it through the day. I took advanced classes and increased my hours at school to be able to only have to attend half days my senior year.

As a freshman, my mom told me about a makeup called Covermark. I was curious, so we went to the department store to check it out. As a young teen whose only goal in life was to be invisible, this was one of the most traumatic days of my adolescence. The girl working the counter pulled a chair into the middle of the walkway of the store and sat me in it. She then proceeded to apply the makeup. This was a long process and required many steps. As she worked, a small crowd formed around me, watching. I could hear the comments and the statements: "Wow, she looks so much better," "I can't imagine living with that on my face," "I am glad she can cover it," and so on.

Internally, I just wanted to be away from there, away from the stares, the comments, all of it. Fighting back tears, I sat in silence, feeling like an even bigger freak as people walking by stared at me. I did end up using the makeup for years.

The process was a nightmare and took up to an hour every morning—applying the thick foundation, putting on the setting powder, and waiting twenty minutes before I could brush off the powder to see if the makeup went on "right." If it did, it was a good day. If it did not, it was a bad day.

My mom was so patient with me and so understanding of how I struggled and how I longed to just be normal. Unfortunately, kids are jerks, no matter what, and I went from being bullied for the birthmark to being bullied for the makeup. One girl looked at me, laughed, and asked me if I applied the makeup with a spackle knife.

I did not really date or even try to date as a teen. My sophomore year, some of the boys made a list of the ugliest girls in school, and they passed it around. Of course, my name was on it. I had the usual crushes. One even told me he liked me a lot; however, he could not ask me out, as his friends would make fun of him. The boyfriends I did have mostly lived in the small town my cousin, who was my best friend, was from, as they tended to be kinder and less judgmental, or I dated college-age men. Regardless, my relationship experience was very minimal.

When I was eighteen, I was doing what we usually did on a Saturday night where I grew up—cruising uptown. Even though I wanted to be invisible, I loved fast cars. A lot. So I bought a Firebird TransAm and could be found most every weekend driving downtown, showing her off, and even at times racing. When I was behind the wheel, I felt powerful and as if I could be myself.

One night, I pulled next to a Porsche, looked over, and locked eyes with who would become my first husband. He was nineteen and cruising with his friends. We exchanged numbers, and the trajectory of my life changed. Initially, the relationship was not bad and certainly not the violent thing it eventually turned into. I was flattered he was interested in me; he was older, in college, came from a well-off family, and had well-off friends. As an eighteen-year-old who grew up in a lower middle-class family, this was a look into a world I had no experience with, and it was amazing to feel included and accepted.

As we dated and the months went by, slowly the relationship changed, and he became more abusive. He began to say hurtful things—for example, I should not complain about anything he did as I should be grateful he loved someone who looked like me; no one else would ever love someone who looked like me. As I shrank smaller and smaller into myself, his abuse grew more and more. We ended up getting married when I was nineteen, and our son was born a year later.

Two years later, I became pregnant with my second son even though my husband had become more and more violent, verbally abusive, and emotionally abusive. He was depriving me of food and sleep, and it was incredibly difficult. He kept saying that I had to take the abuse, no one else would ever love me, I needed to be grateful he tolerated me and to understand how pathetic I was. I lived this life for five years. For me, it took him threatening the lives of my babies to make the final cut and divorce him.

At twenty-three, I found myself a single mother of an almost four-year-old and basically a newborn. Still struggling to find my worth and my value, I simply worked and survived for the next few years. As I aged, the way I saw myself began to change as well. I had worn the Covermark makeup since I was fifteen; when I turned twenty-four, I made the decision to no longer hide behind the mask of makeup and stepped into my adult life for the first time barefaced.

A slight digression from my story—when I was sixteen, my parents learned of a laser being used to treat PWS. At that time (1983-ish), it was very much experimental, and the long-term outcome was unknown. We all talked about it for a bit and made the choice for me to have laser treatment. The laser was an argon laser, and unlike the lasers of today, the point was the size of a pinhead. Basically, they lasered pore by pore. It took about thirty minutes to cover a postage-stamp-sized area. The pain was severe, and no pain mitigation was offered.

I only had one of these treatments as I was severely burned and, to this day, have scar tissue where I was treated. After this initial experience, I was very loath to pursue any more laser treatments; however, when I was around twenty, I learned of a new laser that was less likely to burn. It took less time to administer as well; they could treat the entire birthmark in around twenty minutes. I began these treatments and had around ten before I was no longer able to afford them. This was a PDL.

I believe the doctor also passed with a YAG. This laser gave me good fading, so my self-confidence grew. As it did, so did my voice. I was not trying to date or have a relationship because I was still recovering from the abusive marriage, and providing a stable home for my sons was my priority. At around twenty-four to twenty-five years old, for the first time, I felt as if I was in control of my life and not living a story others had written for me.

As my confidence began to grow, I became braver and bolder. My personality began to emerge, and I discovered I am an extrovert! Well, sometimes, that is. I began to make eye contact with people as I moved through my life, meeting stares with smiles, instead of looking away. Of course, at times it still bothered me. One time in particular stands out. Well, two times.

The first was when I was having high tea at a local teahouse. When the waiter saw my face, he was startled and dropped the tray he was carrying. Another, a woman literally ran into a light pole because she was staring at me so hard.

Even with this, I was able to laugh about it. Living with a facial difference is such a complicated thing. On one hand, we long at times to just look like everyone else. Then, I think of everything my difference has taught me—kindness, compassion, and acceptance. It has taught me to never judge a person based on appearance. It has taught me the worst in people and the best in people. Mostly, it has taught me empathy. Throughout my life, I have been drawn to helping professions such as teaching. For many years, I taught pre-K where my daughter went to school.

After another divorce, I found myself at forty with three children to support and no real way to do so. I returned to college, this time as a graduate student. My focus was clinical psychology, family and child development, and substance-abuse studies. After graduation, I worked with adolescent girls in a residential treatment center, with women in a felon-diversion program working to live a life of sobriety and productivity, as a group facilitator at a retreat center where the work was focused on inner-child healing, and in my position today as executive director of our state's only recovery high school. My firm belief is the empathy I developed for others struggling is rooted in my own experiences of feeling marginalized and outside of the norm.

As a child, kindness and service were ingrained in my brother and me. Our parents worked in missions, my mom teaching English to Hispanic mothers and my father providing laboratory support in the mission's medical unit. My brother and I helped, playing with the children my mom was teaching and helping our dad with organizing. Additionally, we regularly went to the nursing home in our neighborhood. We sang Christmas carols, helped decorate, and read to the residents. All that is to say I was raised in a home where serving others was paramount and showing kindness was the only way. Entering into the world, I had the belief that others were the same, and when I learned that was not the case, it was difficult and painful.

In my life, relationships have been a challenge. I have found myself with men who have used my facial difference as a way to control me, abuse me, and place me in a "less than" position. I have been told by partners more than once I should be grateful they were willing to be with someone who looks like me.

Since divorcing again five years ago, I have learned who I am and have found the strength to set boundaries. At times, those boundaries are respected, and at other times, they are not. What never changes is my knowledge, at my core, of who I am as a person, and I really like the woman I am today. Additionally, I have learned to embrace the inherent beauty in being different. The world is full of imperfections, and those imperfections are what bring beauty to the world.

About two years ago, I got a follow request on Instagram from @mufasapws83, and that request has changed so much of my life for the better. It was from a young man who also lives with a PWS. He had recently found the Vascular Birthmark Foundation, and he was following all the global ambassadors, of which I am one. We began to message and chat, and we immediately became friends. During that time, he lost a parent and began adjusting to his new life. We chatted often, offering support and sometimes just a listening presence.

Through Adrian, I have been connected to so many others in the birthmark community, including the people in this anthology. Connecting to others like me has been truly incredible and life-changing. I wish so much these groups had been around when I was growing up so I could have known I was not alone. The gratitude I have that these groups and support options are available today is immeasurable. Knowing other children and adolescents navigating life with a difference have a community to provide love and support…it is just the best.

Through my connection to Adrian, last summer I had the incredible gift of meeting several others in the birthmark community. We all sat at a table in La Jolla, California, with the ocean as a backdrop, and I realized it was the first time in my entire life I was sitting at a table at which I was not the different one. None of us was different because we were all together. We shared stories, struggles, triumphs, joys, sadnesses, our experiences with laser treatments, and how the public interacts with us. We laughed a lot, and we also shed tears. Most of all, we simply connected with people who truly understood; that was the greatest gift. What I took away from that day was the importance of community, connection, and acceptance. My hope is I will be able to experience much more of this.

Thinking of the past, compared to today, I have nothing but hope for the generations coming behind me. The importance of promoting facial equality and combating the view perpetuated by the media and entertainment industry that facial differences are somehow inherently evil or malevolent cannot be understated. Fear is learned. Education is the key to acceptance.

I want to encourage the younger generation to keep fighting for equality and to take up space in the world. You are light bringers, hope dealers, and inclusion warriors! For me, I am excited to be a part of this movement and a voice for others.

Some days are easier than others; some days, I still question my worth and if I will ever be loved for myself, complications and all. But at the core, I am comfortable in my skin for the first time in my life.

To conclude, as I review all the experiences my birthmark has brought me, overall, I am still grateful. Full transparency—if someone came to me today and said they could take the birthmark away, I would no doubt be tempted. But I do not think I would take them up on the offer. My birthmark made me, me, and I like who I am. I like the person I became. I have no regrets for loving whom I loved and for trying to find my own person to love me. My reflection and I have become friends. I like how the red of my birthmark highlights my green eyes. I like how one of my cheeks is a little fuller than the other. I like finding opportunities to educate others on tolerance and kindness. Most of all, I like this community of love and friendship we have built.

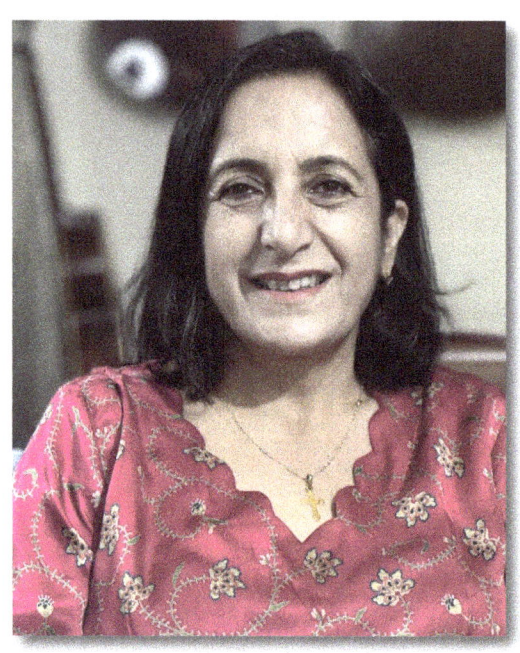

"As I scanned the room in a panic, a nurse walked in with a small burrito of towels. It was my baby! I had achieved the impossible."

# DEATH KNOCKED ON MY DOOR ELEVEN TIMES

*Batool Kaushal*

I didn't know what Klippel-Trenaunay syndrome (KTS) was until I was forty. When I finally got to name the condition that defined my life, I had more than a story to tell, but for now, this is my KTS story.

I was born in a middle-class Muslim family in a small village in Kashmir, India. Born as a twin, my brother left me soon after coming into this world. At eighteen months, my parents saw I was passing fresh blood in my stools. The doctors treated me for hemorrhoids. My parents left no stone unturned for my treatment, yet I continued to bleed. By my fourth birthday, I had been under the knife four times in Kashmir, at a time when specialized medicine in India was in its primal stages.

I welcomed my teenage years with pain and varicose veins stretching across my right leg. Every doctor advised crepe bandages and iron supplements. I soon had a limp. My right leg was growing slightly longer than the left leg with the veins bulging out. At the same time, the frequent bleeding caused my hemoglobin to plummet from five to four pints.

My brushes with death became an everyday affair, and my chances for survival were slim. My mother fed me homemade pomegranate juice every day to maintain my hemoglobin.

It wasn't until my father took a leap of faith and flew me to the Postgraduate Institute of Medical Sciences and Research in Chandigarh for treatment.

We went straight from the airport to the emergency room, where my hemoglobin test screamed a low three pints. The retest came in at three pints again. The doctor was surprised I could walk normally. Medically, I should have been dead or in intensive care.

The ER is an eerie place of wails, cries, trauma, and blood. Too scary a scenario for a teenager to be thrown into. I refused to get admitted to an emergency ward and ran out into the hallway.

With no place to go, my father met other Kashmiris, and the only place they found near the hospital was a car park that turned into a dormitory at night. We camped there. I was a young girl in an unknown place at night, strangers sleeping all around me on the ground; my father was up all night keeping watch.

The next morning, I was admitted into the gastroenterology department. For the next three months, my world revolved around patients, attendants, nurses, and doctors while my classmates were finishing their senior year of high school.

I was given six pints of blood in two weeks. Two months later, when the medical testing was complete, a general surgeon with his team of doctors started working on the modalities for performing a life-threatening or life-altering surgery on me. I was told the chance of survival was only one percent. One day before the surgery, I told my dad, "I don't think I am going to die."

On January 18, 1981, at 7:00 a.m., I was wheeled into the operating room. The doctor placed a black anesthesia mask on my face, and I went into a deep slumber. I was dreaming of riding golden horses in green pastures. According to one nurse, my intestines were being repaired on one table and my body on the other, laced with tubes and pipes, but my brain was actively enjoying the most beautiful images.

After the eight-hour surgery, I woke up in the recovery room. I heard my father's shaky voice as he asked, "How are you, Batool?"

Still groggy from the anesthesia, I simply asked for the time.

The attending surgeon jokingly asked, "Hey, Batool, you want to go for a walk?"

I lost consciousness again, but… Oh. My. God. I was alive!

Two weeks later, I was ready to fly home with a colostomy bag. During the eighties in India, it was taboo for a young girl to have health problems. So my father decided not to reveal the colostomy bag tied to my belly to anyone, not even my mother. He cleaned it every day. When my aunts asked to see the surgical scar on my belly, I brushed it off with an excuse.

The sight of a temporary stoma (opening) on my stomach was very scary, and I wanted it closed at the earliest opportunity. Three months later, another surgery brought an end to the stoma and cleaning of the colostomy bag, but for another three months, I had to be on a liquid diet. Even that, though, felt refreshing.

As it is in most Indian communities, my family, though skeptical, still pursued marriage proposals for me. My mother wished for me to marry a healthy man, but it was difficult for any man to accept me with my KTS, so I discarded the idea of marriage for the next thirteen years. My KTS leg had its moments of trouble, but largely life was good. I was excelling on my career path to be an academic and was set to start a research program at Oxford University in the United Kingdom.

It all came crashing down on a sleepy Sunday afternoon. Mild constipation triggered my internal KTS, and I bled profusely from both the uterine wall and intestines. This continued until late at night. I was alone in my apartment, and as advised by my surgeon, I elevated my legs and lay motionless on the bed. The bleeding subsided, but it didn't stop. According to the surgeon, these types of recurrences were possible.

I called the landlady. She stood in utter shock and disbelief, urging me to go to a gynecologist for what she assumed was a miscarriage. She looked around the blood-splattered floor and called her housekeeper to clean it up. I managed to get through the night.

The next morning, I regained some strength and was able to get to the hospital. After examining me, the doctor simply advised me to consult my surgeon at PGI Chandigarh. By the time my family was informed, my cousin was there to help me board a bus to Chandigarh. I could sense eyes on me in the bus; a man sitting in the front row had noticed me. The bus stopped at a service station, and this man approached me to ask if I was from Kashmir. He introduced himself as Major Kaushal from the Indian army. I am not one for unnecessary conversations with strangers, but I kept on with the small talk. He must have noticed my frail condition, as he offered to drop me off at my accommodations. I wasn't in a position to decline.

The next day, my brother arrived, and we met with the surgeon who was in shock and advised an immediate angiogram. My entire pelvis was full of blood, and the radiologists could not identify the source of the bleeding. The surgeon asked for a follow-up examination in two weeks, but he looked increasingly uncertain about my survival.

In the midst of chaos, the major I met on the bus called and visited me in the hospital. Preoccupied with my health, I couldn't even remember if I had given him my contact number.

Meanwhile, my surgeon suggested a plan for my treatment:

> First, hormone therapy.
>
> Next, if that didn't work, embolization of the bleeding vessels.
>
> Finally, if that didn't work either, surgery, which was again the life-threatening and life-altering option.

With these suggestions, the surgeon referred me to the All India Institute of Medical Sciences at Delhi. There I met a renowned gynecologist who advised hormone therapy, and within four days, the bleeding stopped. The monthly ultrasound of my pelvis showed that the KTS was shrinking. It was a relief beyond measure. Finally, something had worked! I had long accepted the fate that KTS had no cure, but knowing that it was treatable, I was ecstatic.

The army major visited me and kept track of my health. We began dating, and, randomly during a coffee date, he proposed to me.

I laughed and said, "You are mad. I am going to die."

He wasn't one to back down. He walked straight into my doctor's office and asked if he could marry me.

The doctor smiled and said, "Sure, but don't have kids; I won't be able to save her then."

Another year passed, and we got married.

The hormone therapy brought another reality. I was thirty-five, and I wanted to have kids. With the KTS internally across my abdomen and externally straining my leg, I knew pregnancy would be difficult, but the hormone therapy that was making life livable put a full stop to conception. I was at a crossroads. Do I fulfill my wish of becoming a mother or enjoy the now-manageable KTS?

The first conception ended in a miscarriage. I couldn't bear it, so I decided to take a risk. I stopped taking the hormone pill. Soon, I conceived. My husband and I were happy but anxious. To carry on with the pregnancy was too risky, but I wanted to keep the baby. Throughout the pregnancy, my gynecologist and vascular surgeon were sitting on speed dial.

At four months, I had a small episode of bleeding. My husband and I panicked. The fetus was growing and needed space, thus straining internal organs and the KTS. Further along, the pregnancy went smoothly.

I couldn't bear the thought of my baby suffering my same ordeal. Like any mother, I wanted to be assured that my baby had no vascular irregularities in her body. The gynecologist scheduled an elective classical cesarean on March 31, 2000. I was admitted to Sitaram Bhartia Institute of Science and Research in Delhi. At 7:00 a.m., I was placed on a gurney and taken into the operating room.

Before the surgery, the gynecologist asked my husband, "Worst-case scenario, who do you want us to save, the mother or the baby?"

He replied, "BOTH."

Under general anesthesia, I was out cold. I woke up with severe pain in my lower abdomen. *Is the surgery over? Where is my baby?* As I scanned the room in a panic, a nurse walked in with a small burrito of towels. It was my baby!

"Congratulations, you are blessed with a baby girl," said the nurse.

I had achieved the impossible. The baby was premature and needed neonatal care; otherwise, she was completely healthy. My husband and I couldn't believe it. Our prayers had been answered, and it was worth the risk.

We thoroughly enjoyed parenthood, watching our girl grow, but my KTS bled off and on. The doctor repeatedly put me on hormone therapy. It was frustrating; there was only so much my body could handle postpartum.

A friend suggested pranic healing. I wasn't a very spiritual person, but I gave it a try. After twenty-five healings, suddenly at night I was sweating, vomiting, urinating, and defecating—all at once. I felt as if I were going to die. After such a deep cleansing of my body, I felt very light. I don't know if it was a divine intervention, the medications, or the pranic healing, but my KTS went back to a manageable state.

Fourteen years passed, and life was good with routine medical interventions. My little baby grew into a beautiful young girl. While she was studying at a British boarding school and my husband was working abroad, I lived alone and worked. To spend some time with my husband, I traveled to Bhutan. Little did I know that would put me back where I started.

A few days into the trip, severe pain appeared in my KTS leg. We were in the middle of nowhere in the countryside of Bhutan, where for miles there was not even a living soul, let alone a hospital. The pain grew unbearable, and no painkillers or home remedies provided any relief. The airport was a twelve-hour drive, but we had no choice but to make the tedious road journey. En route, the agonizing pain made me lose my senses briefly.

We rushed from the airport to the military hospital and consulted a vascular surgeon, who did prescribe a few medications. The medicine had the least effect on my leg. I was again shuffling from one hospital to another. Actually, no doctor could diagnose and treat my problem.

I resorted to Googling my symptoms. After going down a couple of internet rabbit holes, I found the Vascular Birthmarks Foundation (VBF). I contacted VBF's president and founder, Dr. Linda-Rozell Shannon. She led me to New York City's Lenox Hill Hospital, and an interventional radiologist there agreed to operate on my leg. After the shortest surgery ever done on my KTS, I was lying in the recovery room of Lenox Hill Hospital with my leg wrapped in bandages. First time ever I could see the lower part of my leg without bulging blue veins and without pain. When I returned to India, I was back at the gym, and I was at my healthiest.

As a KTS patient, being at your healthiest doesn't negate the need for routine screenings. A routine ultrasound showed a cyst rapidly growing in my right ovary. By the end of 2014, the cyst was eleven centimeters. I could feel it when I touched my belly. Cutting me open wasn't an easy option, as the ovaries were surrounded by dense vascularity.

"Can you find a laparoscopic surgeon for this? I don't want to do an open surgery because your ovary is surrounded by thick vascularity. It is a high risk," said my gynecologist.

From one referral to another, this time I landed in a laparoscopic surgeon's office in Mumbai at Breach Candy Hospital. Each day, my anxiety was growing alongside the cyst. *What if the cyst bursts? Is this going to be another near-death experience?* This was an unexpected diagnosis not related to my KTS. KTS was my life, and I had started loving it. According to one surgeon, being cut open several times could have caused the cyst, or it could have been the hormone pill.

The doctors at Breach Candy formed a team of nine specialists to be present during surgery, including a vascular surgeon and a surgical oncologist. Fortunately, the cyst was benign and was removed. However, this recovery was different from those after my KTS surgeries. I spent ten days in the hospital, and even though I was feeling too weak, the surgeon advised me to go home.

Back home, my condition deteriorated. Possibly, the high doses of antibiotics and painkillers had activated the bleeding in my intestinal vasculature. I was in pain and bedridden. My husband had to carry me from the bed to the toilet.

I was back on the Ferris wheel of multiple consultations. Each doctor left to return to their textbooks whenever I described my medical history. This time, a Padma Shri gastroenterologist was brave enough to take a chance on me. He put me on a liquid diet for seven days to prepare me for a double GI endoscopy under general anesthesia. One day before the procedure, I defecated in my pants while entering the hospital. I was embarrassed, but my husband cleaned me. He was always unconditional in his care. The gastroenterologist closed the leaks in my intestinal KTS with a laser. He warned me about becoming constipated and wrote a prescription for high-dose laxatives.

As with most of the world, all was fine until COVID. More than a year passed without any medical checkups, even though I was having issues with my digestive system—bloating, acidity, sleeplessness, mouth blisters, and a few kilos of weight loss. I consulted my gynecologist online, who again prescribed hormone therapy and postmenopausal supplements.

At this juncture, something unusual and alarming was happening in my body. I was feeling a hard-stabbing streak on one side of my left breast. Masked up, I managed to get to the military hospital.

After the examination, the surgeon asked me, "Where do you want me to refer you to, Delhi or Mumbai?"

My suspicions were confirmed. It definitely wasn't KTS related, but it was equally frightening.

Soon, I was at Medanta Hospital in Delhi. Three days after a biopsy, the breast surgeon wanted to operate on me as soon as possible. I was agitated. *Another surgery?* But this time it was stage 2 breast cancer. *Is it the result of postmenopausal hormone therapy?* Fearless me thought, *If I can handle KTS for fifty-seven years, I can fight this too.*

So I had emergency breast surgery. In recovery, the surgeon came running to me and said, "Good news is, it is out; bad news, it was in one of the lymph nodes, therefore this drain."

To the hospital staff, I was the easiest patient to handle because I was very familiar with medical procedures and devices. Due to the huge influx of COVID patients, I was discharged the same day from the hospital.

The world of surgery, both in and out of operating rooms, was my territory; however, this postoperative recovery followed by chemo and radiation gave me jitters. But I kept my head up. The first of six cycles of chemotherapy began, and it hit me like a boulder. Side effects—from vomiting to stinking breath—mounted, not to mention the shedding of hair.

The hospital had been my playground as a chronically ill child, but as a chemo recipient, I loathed it. My husband and I spent our twenty-fifth wedding anniversary in the hospital. There was a deafening silence in the room as we tearfully wished each other many more.

Each chemo round grew in intensity. At the second cycle of chemo, it felt as if I were losing the battle. My husband prayed and asked me to do the same. The nurse kept injecting the IV drip. I was in a semiconscious state when I felt the hands of

Jesus Christ hovering over my body and His robes touching me, assuring me of my complete recovery. When I woke up, I felt light and blessed.

Finally, six cycles of chemo were over, and a month of radiology treatments started immediately. This yearlong treatment altered my brain chemistry. It was the most excruciating and disturbing period of my life. I had become too weak physically and too agitated mentally. In remission, I was put on an initial five-year plan to take one Letrozole tablet every day to keep the cancer away.

Here, after three years, words are failing me when attempting to address the scars from the battles already won. I made lifestyle changes, increased my workout regimen, and expanded my social circles. It improved my physical health, and I became a "glass half full" person.

Death came knocking horrendously several times in my sixty-one years of life, but I kept the door shut to write my story.

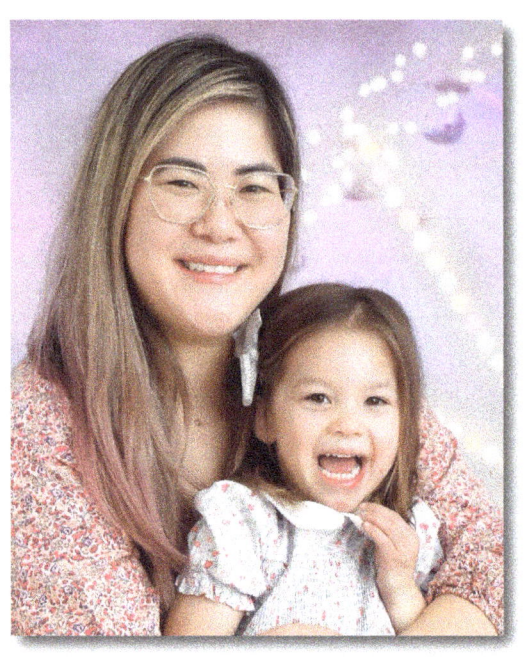

"Since her birth, we'd always addressed her birthmark, to her and others, with a matter-of-fact and casual attitude. It is simply just part of her, another uniquely beautiful characteristic that makes her the wonderful person she is."

# AMAZING AMELIA
## Crystal Gordon

*From the moment you were born,
you became the sun to my planet.*

—*Author unknown*

For nine months, we happily planned for and anticipated the moment we would meet our baby. I remember, during my second trimester, the doctor's office called us to go over our genetics screening, which was reported as completely normal, and to share with us that our baby was a girl. We were overjoyed to find out we were having a girl! My husband was so ecstatic that he ran a few laps around the room.

With each passing month, her kicks grew stronger in my belly, and we became more eager to become parents. We cherished every opportunity we got to see her during ultrasounds, especially since I was pregnant during the COVID pandemic, and restrictions were being strictly enforced.

My husband and I excitedly welcomed our sweet baby girl, Amelia, into this world on a perfect spring evening. She was absolutely beautiful and perfect in every way! As soon as the nurse laid her on top of me, I looked at her adorable, tiny face, then immediately grabbed her itsy-bitsy fingers and toes. As I held her for the first time, I vaguely remember the nurse quickly and nonchalantly mentioning something about her having a birthmark. But our daughter, Amelia, had finally arrived, and I was solely focused on soaking in every second of it!

About a couple of minutes later, one of the delivery nurses came to me, pulled her face mask down, and said while smiling, "She has a birthmark like me!" My brain did not register exactly what she meant since I was still dazed from having just gone through the experience of giving birth minutes before, and at the time, I wasn't at all familiar with what a vascular birthmark was. I had waited all that time to meet my beloved baby, and nothing else mattered in that moment except holding her and being with her.

In the hours that followed, we found out she had a port-wine stain (PWS) birthmark. The birthmark covered part of her scalp and extended down over her ear, eye, cheek, chin, and part of her neck. At that point, we didn't even have time to consider the birthmark since the hospital whisked her away to admit her to the NICU for jaundice. She remained in the NICU for two days, and during that time, we noticed one of the NICU doctors also had a facial port-wine stain. Statistically, three in every one thousand babies are born with a port-wine stain, so what were the chances we would encounter two adults who had port-wine stains within the first couple of days after Amelia's birth? It was definitely reassuring to have had these encounters and experiences with these medical professionals at the time, especially since neither my husband nor I had ever heard of and were not familiar with port-wine stains and vascular birthmarks.

While we were in the hospital for the duration of her NICU stay, my husband spearheaded researching everything he could about port-wine stains. He was our champion and read everything diligently and conveyed it to me so we could prepare and plan for what we could do to best support our daughter.

Using the recommendations of the hospital and doctors, we agreed there were three priorities. The most important thing we wanted to evaluate was her susceptibility to seizures, which are common with Sturge-Weber syndrome (SWS), a condition that sometimes manifests with facial port-wine stains. Next, we wanted to monitor her risk of glaucoma since her port-wine stain is near her eye.

Finally, we wanted to consult with specialists who could perform laser therapy to help keep her skin healthy around her PWS. If left untreated the skin where the PWS is could thicken, become larger and darker, and develop bumps and blebs. Studies show that consistent and frequent exposure to pulsed-dye laser therapy earlier in life is highly effective in achieving clear skin. Although, it should be noted that clearing up the PWS one hundred percent was not likely, even with the pulsed-dye laser therapy. However, clear skin was never the goal for us personally; we just wanted to keep her skin healthy.

A lot of our research findings were derived from medical websites, and we were lucky to stumble across the extremely positive and supportive vascular-birthmark community on Instagram and Facebook. Searching Instagram using @portwinestain and joining the Facebook groups Port-Wine Stain Birthmarks, To Treat or Not to Treat and Birthmark, and Port-Wine Stain Family and Friends, we found so many individual and family contacts who were willing to share their experiences and support!

In retrospect, there were so many reassuring moments about Amelia's PWS throughout her first few weeks of life that I do not recall many lingering moments of anxiety or fear, which understandably many first-time parents would feel. I really was confident that with our knowledge and resources, we would be able to do whatever we needed to give our daughter the best care.

Eventually, Amelia's jaundice subsided, and we were allowed to return home with her. The following weeks were a flurry of blissfully blurry memories typical of bringing home a newborn. She was thriving and growing stronger every day. She loved her milk and being held. I loved holding her while lovingly gazing into her entrancing, large gray eyes. She was our Amazing Amelia and the biggest joy in our lives every day!

When introducing our newest bundle of joy to our friends and family, everyone seemed just as captivated as we were with her lovable nature. Of course, the topic of her PWS came up, but it was more out of curiosity since it seemed as though no one knew about vascular birthmarks. We would simply say, "It's her birthmark!" and give some basic facts about PWS. Everyone—and I mean everyone—was understanding and interested. We couldn't take her out of the house without getting compliments about how adorable she was.

In her first few weeks, she was already teaching us so much! As most parents know firsthand, children can be great life teachers who help us learn more about ourselves and the world around us. We were, and will always be, so lucky to have her and she, us.

In trying to find specialists who best fit us and our needs, there were certain challenges. The first was finding that our city severely lacked the specialists we needed. Thankfully, to monitor her risk of glaucoma, we were able to secure care from the only pediatric optometrist in our town. We see her for annual screenings. We were also able to make an appointment with one of the few pediatric neurologists in town; he performed an electroencephalogram (EEG) to rule out any brain activity associated with seizures, which are often caused by SWS.

Then it came time to find a laser specialist who could help treat Amelia's PWS. Unfortunately, not only were there no specialists in town we trusted with this delicate procedure, but also we ran into an insurance issue. We expanded our search to nearby major cities in other states and eventually found two specialists we were comfortable with, but our insurance would not cover the out-of-state visits. We felt strongly about seeing these out-of-state doctors, so we switched our insurance. If you are familiar with the American healthcare system, that is not an easy process. After a couple of months of back-and-forth insurance discussions, we were able to receive care from Dr. John Stuart Nelson at the UCI Beckman Laser Institute in Irvine, California.

The treatment plan at first was aggressive—every two weeks. Trips to Dr. Nelson were rough, to say the least. Traveling with an infant every two weeks for medical day trips was mentally, emotionally, physically, and financially exhausting for us all. My husband and I were lucky enough to be able to manage these trips and gladly made them because we knew we were giving our daughter the best care.

Eventually, the treatment intervals lengthened to every four weeks, and then every two months. Around that time, we became aware that the treatments did not result in clearance of the PWS. *Clearance* is the term doctors use to describe the reduction of the visible redness and size of the vascular birthmark. The doctor believed additional treatments at the two-month range were not going to provide any more clearance, so he advised that we return every four months for maintenance treatments to keep her skin healthy. This was a huge relief to us.

Around her eighteenth treatment, we hit another roadblock with insurance. Even though this insurance company had paid for seventeen prior treatments, they declined to cover any in the future. They deemed these ongoing treatments as cosmetic and not medically necessary. We pursued the appeal process for multiple months, which included a lot of back-and-forth, peer-to-peer conversations between the insurance company and Dr. Nelson's office. The insurance company denied our appeal even after our doctor's conversation with their medical director.

I was not going to give up without a fight and was determined to get my daughter's treatments covered, as I not only wanted her to receive the best care but also because I truly believe they are medically necessary, not something we are doing for cosmetic reasons.

Our next option was to submit an internal appeal, which meant writing a letter to detail why the denial should be overturned and providing clinical documentation to prove the procedures were medically necessary. I spent about a month gathering all the materials I would need to write a thorough appeal. It included the following:

- A letter of medical necessity for this treatment from her provider, Dr. Nelson

- Five peer-reviewed research articles from published medical journals

- The American Academy of Pediatrics vascular-anomalies letter of medical necessity (https://birthmark.org/insurance-claims/)

- Before and after photos of my child

I found a template for the appeal letter on the Vascular Birthmark Foundation's website, under their Insurance Claims and Appeals tab, and started writing. I feverishly worked on the letter for about a week or two. My finalized appeal packet was forty pages long, which included all the materials I referenced. In my letter, I pleaded with them to carefully read the factual information I provided and reevaluate their decision. I mailed the packet off and waited to hear back.

It took a couple of weeks to hear back, and when I did, they told me they would take another month or so to review the case. While we were waiting, we did not want Amelia to stop receiving her treatments, so we ended up paying for two treatments out of our own pockets. The University of California was in charge of billing since Dr. Nelson's office is part of their Beckman Laser Institute. They offered us a cash price which was thousands of dollars per treatment. We were able to continue by using a credit card.

We eventually heard back from our insurance company; our appeal was finally approved! Additionally, they were going to retroactively pay for the two treatments we paid for out of pocket. That reimbursement process took a whole additional year and was excruciatingly frustrating; however, I was still grateful that the costs were covered. I felt as though my persistence had paid off, and I was glad I had done it.

We have since had another denial, once again deeming the procedures cosmetic, but it was quickly overturned during the peer-to-peer conversation they had with Dr. Nelson. I anticipate it won't be our last insurance issue regarding Amelia's PWS treatments, and I am prepared to deal with it as it comes.

A common parenthood cliche is that your little one's childhood passes too quickly. In retrospect, we truly didn't understand what that meant—or more likely, how that felt—until we experienced it as parents. With infancy and toddlerhood behind her, which really did seem as if it passed in a blink of an eye, Amelia was poised to start pre-K. Amelia is extremely bright, curious, social, and well-spoken, so we were very excited for her to be in an environment that would help her grow not only academically but also socially.

Coupled with our excitement over her starting school was our anxiety about how her new classmates would react and treat her because of her PWS. I think parents naturally worry about their children, but I was an elementary school teacher for a number of years, so I saw firsthand how bullying impacts children. However, I also know that there are so many positively beautiful experiences and memories that can occur within a school setting. We didn't want to shield her from the world, but I knew we needed to arm her with the support, skills, and tools to face the world confidently.

Since her birth, we'd always addressed her birthmark, to her and others, with a matter-of-fact and casual attitude. It is simply just part of her, another uniquely beautiful characteristic that makes her the wonderful person she is. Unfortunately, there is a negative stigma associated with vascular birthmarks, or more generally with anything that deviates from the social norms of beauty.

Therefore, I knew it was critical for us to help her not just feel beautiful on the outside but also feel confident from within as well. We helped her find her inner confidence by encouraging her success in developmentally appropriate activities and extracurricular activities, such as dancing and swimming. We celebrated her perseverance and hard work whenever she succeeded in something she was working hard on, focusing on the effort put in as well as the results.

She developed a lot of determination, and we are always happy to let her try new things, with guidance and support where we see appropriate. When she was about a year and half years old, I started reading her children's books about birthmarks. Our favorites are *Sam's Birthmark* by Martha and Grant Griffin and *Made Marvelous* by Adree Williams.

Around the same time, another mom in our city, Hila, reached out to me to connect because her child has a very similar PWS. We have playdates, and I deeply value our connection and believe it's important for our children to have someone else they can relate to on this level.

Amelia became pretty comfortable with her PWS, so much so that one day, when she saw a random woman at the park, one with a PWS, she went up to her and said, "You have a birthmark just like me; we match!"

By the time she started school at three years old, she had the verbal skills of a five- or six-year-old. To prepare her for school socially, we equipped her with phrases to use as responses in certain situations. These phrases ranged from "No, thank you, I don't want to play right now" to "Oh, this is just my birthmark; it's pink, like my favorite color." It provided *her* with confidence because she had the tools to face new situations, and it provided *us* with comfort, knowing she felt prepared. An unexpected positive effect of this is that now she is comfortable coming to us to ask us what she should say or do in situations when she is unsure how to respond.

Four months into the school year, she was due for a laser treatment, which would leave her with visible and dark bruising all over the treated area. Amelia was already used to her purple dots—what we call the bruising—but I knew her classmates were not. I wanted to introduce the class to the concept and asked the teacher if I could be a guest reader and read *Made Marvelous*. Her teacher was very welcoming, as inclusion and celebrating each other's differences are things that are valued in her school.

In addition to reading the book, I wanted to emphasize to the class how we are all unique and different. Amelia is comfortable talking about her birthmark, so she was happy to share more about it. I also spent time discussing some of my unique features and asked the other children to do the same. It was a very positive experience all around, and I felt pretty good about how it was received.

After Amelia returned to school with her purple dots, she relayed that no one really seemed to comment on them. Surprisingly, she actually seemed a little let down by the underwhelming reaction of her classmates because she wanted to show them off! It really makes my mommy heart proud and happy to know she is so comfortable and confident about herself.

Parenthood has been an interesting nonstop ride filled with transformative lessons and profound core memories. I am so grateful for my husband who is the best partner. I am so proud of my daughter, my Amazing Amelia, who is as confidently fierce as she is kind and sweet. I know, together as a family, we will work to do our best to overcome any challenges we may face. All we can do is take it one day at a time and do the best we can with what we have.

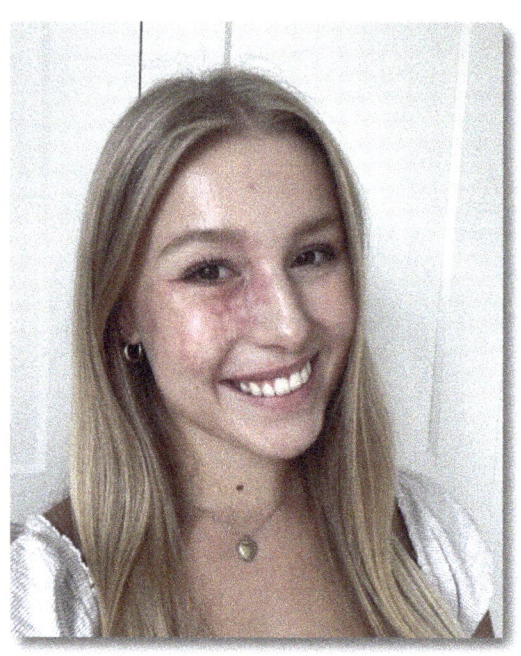

"This is not a story about a bullied girl. This is a story about how my facial difference helped me grow into a stronger person and build unshakable confidence."

# A SHORT STORY ABOUT CONFIDENCE

*Dana Marie Rückert*

"What's that on your face?"

"Ew, you have such bad acne!"

"I'm so sorry for you—did you burn your face?!"

I have a facial difference. A port-wine stain. Sometimes, I even forget about it. To be honest, having a port-wine stain has shaped my upbringing in many ways. Even after my best friend in elementary school told me that I looked like a monster, I never dared to lose my confidence. I knew I was not going to let my port-wine stain alone define me.

My parents always reminded me that my birthmark was just a part—a very special one—of me, but not a flaw. Growing up, I learned to use humor as a tool to navigate people's reactions. But this is not a story about a bullied girl. This is a story about how my facial difference helped me grow into a stronger person and build unshakable confidence.

Let me start at the beginning. From what my parents told me, I know some things about my early years. When they received my diagnosis—their daughter had a port-wine stain—they were scared. Understandably so. If I were having my first child with a facial difference, I would likely be concerned as well. After extensive research, they decided that I should receive pulsed-dye laser treatment early on.

My first laser surgery was at just six weeks old. My mom remembers that it was torture for them to see me like that. During my first treatments, the doctors did not use anesthesia, so my parents had to hold me still. Some might call that cruel, but I am grateful for their decision to be brave and get me treatment.

## THE FIRST TIME I NOTICED MY DIFFERENCE

The first time I realized that I had a facial difference was in a gas-station restroom with my mom. I was about three years old, and we were on our way home after a laser treatment. In the stall, I caught my reflection in the toilet-paper holder. My face had already turned dark purple from the procedure. I started crying and begged my mom to wash off whatever was on my face.

Even though I cannot recall my thoughts, I must have been incredibly confused and could not understand why my face looked bruised and unfamiliar. Panic must have risen in my chest as I struggled to recognize myself.

How do you explain to a three-year-old that their face will not just "wash off"? My mom had already told me about the laser treatments, but, naturally, I wasn't able to grasp what they meant.

## WHAT IS A PORT-WINE STAIN?

A port-wine stain is a capillary malformation in the skin. The swollen blood vessels give it its characteristic red color. Most people have them on their head and neck; mine is on the right side of my face.

But how would I explain this to a child? When I was younger and my peers asked me about my port-wine stain, I would say, "It's like blushing, but all the time," or something like that. I won't bore you with too many scientific facts, but I do want to say that I do not have Sturge-Weber syndrome, a neurological condition sometimes associated with port-wine stains. I'm sure someone else in this book will explain that better than I can.

However, I do experience higher pressure on my optic nerve, which my doctors monitor closely. So far, there has been no damage. Due to the increased blood flow on the right side of my face, that side has grown slightly larger than the left. In a way, it sounds like a superpower. Right now, it doesn't bother me.

## LASER TREATMENT AND ITS IMPACT ON MY LIFE

I mentioned laser therapy earlier, but let me explain what it meant for me. Fortunately, my parents sought treatment when I was only weeks old. The younger you start pulsed-dye laser treatment, the better the chances of lightening the birthmark. So if a parent of a child with a port-wine stain is reading this, I encourage you to pursue treatment early rather than waiting for the child to decide later.

I've lost count of how many laser surgeries I've had over the years. When I was younger, I had several a year, each time under anesthesia. The doctors lasered my entire port-wine stain up to three times per session. Nowadays, I have treatment twice a year in winter, without numbing cream or anesthesia, and they only apply the laser once.

The laser feels as if an elastic band were snapping against your skin; each pulse delivers a sharp sting. Around the nose and mouth, it is especially uncomfortable due to the cooling air used during the procedure. You have to close your eyes because the laser can damage your eyesight. Because of this risk, they can't go too close to my eye, but they still come close enough that I can see the laser light through my eyelid.

Oh, and there is the smell of burnt skin or hair, which isn't exactly pleasant. One time, a doctor accidentally fried some of my eyelashes while using the laser near my eye. It took weeks to grow them back.

After a few pulses, they usually ask if you need a break, but I always tell them to continue as fast as possible. It is not the most comfortable situation, as you can imagine. After treatment, my port-wine stain turns dark purple, kind of like a bruise, and swells up a lot. When I was a kid, I made up jokes to explain it when people asked. I'd say, "I won a boxing match—you should see the other guy!" because the swelling made one of my eyes look way smaller, as if I'd been in a fight. The purple fades back to its usual red after about two weeks, and the swelling goes down in three days.

## RECOVERING FROM LASER THERAPY

After each treatment, I usually spend some time in the city… without makeup. The stares don't bother me as much anymore because I like to believe that people in the city know there's a laser clinic nearby and can figure out what happened. One time, someone wished me a fast recovery because she knew about the clinic, which made me smile.

Do you cover up your pimples with makeup? Funny enough, I do too…but I don't cover up my birthmark. It's a normal part of my face. That changes, however, when my port-wine stain is healing after laser treatment.

*You look like a clown* is a thought I sometimes have when covering up the purple. Sitting there for nearly an hour just to do my base, layering on makeup, correcting colors, adding powder—it just doesn't feel natural. No one should feel the need to paint a mask on their face. And the worst part? People might still stare and wonder why I'm wearing such heavy makeup. *Don't touch your face! I need to check my makeup in the mirror!* These thoughts constantly run through my head. When my port-wine stain is still healing, I don't leave the house without makeup.

I have a theory about this. Let's say you usually have perfect skin, but one day you get a rash. You'd probably cover it up. I normally don't feel the need to cover my birthmark (which is often mistaken for a rash), but when it's bruised and swollen, I do. It's funny how that works.

## PUBLIC PERCEPTION AND CURIOSITY

After my treatments, I always go shopping with my mom. It became a little tradition during my childhood—a reward for being brave. I also walk around with an ice pack on my face. LOL. You should see the stares I get. But I don't judge people for it. If I saw someone walking around with an ice pack on their face, I'd probably wonder what happened too.

Last year, a store manager approached me, concerned, and asked if I needed help. It was a kind gesture, but these are the moments when I feel misunderstood. I don't want people to misinterpret my condition.

This brings me to an important point. I want people to ask me about it. I don't mind the stares, but I care more about people understanding what a port-wine stain is. It's not about attention—I just want people to be informed. There's nothing wrong with curiosity, but there is something wrong with misinterpretation and rude stares.

My mom taught me an important lesson when I was younger. One summer day at the local pool, I saw a boy around my age with no legs. Yet he was climbing up the diving board and jumping off. I stared for a while before finally asking my mom what his condition was. She didn't know but encouraged me to go up to him and ask.

She was right. I approached him, and he was happy to explain his story. He told me that he preferred when people asked questions rather than just stare. That moment stuck with me, and, today, I say the same thing.

## GROWING UP WITH CONFIDENCE

Luckily, I never had real issues because of my birthmark. I grew up in the same town my whole life, so people were used to seeing me. My parents played a huge role in shaping my confidence. They always told me that curiosity was normal, but how I responded to it was up to me. They helped me prepare for the common questions I'd get and even encouraged me to joke about my port-wine stain.

"What if someone asks if you got burned?" my mom would say.

I'd grin and reply, "Nope! Fire mark just sounds cooler!"

Humor quickly became my best way to handle awkward situations. I even came up with a little game. Whenever people stared at me, I'd suddenly say, "Boo!" It worked every time.

Meeting new people has never really intimidated me. In fact, I often forget that my port-wine stain is something unusual to others. But sometimes, I do wonder if people would treat me differently if I didn't have it.

When I was sixteen, I spent ten months in the US as a high school exchange student. Before leaving, I was worried. What if no host family wanted to accommodate me because of my birthmark? But I didn't have to worry for long because just a month after submitting my application, a family was found for me.

I was beyond excited about the adventure ahead and curious about how people would treat me in a completely new environment. To my surprise, I met my best friends on my very first day of school. My worries about how people would react to my looks faded almost immediately. Of course, there were always a few people who seemed more reserved around me, maybe unsure of what to say. But that's their issue, not mine—and that's okay.

I can't force people to be more open, but I try to break the ice if I sense my port-wine stain has become the elephant in the room. Casually mentioning it in conversation has helped more than once.

## ROMANTIC RELATIONSHIPS AND CONFIDENCE

Confidence isn't just about how you see yourself; it also affects how you connect with others. When I was younger, I sometimes wondered how the birthmark would influence romantic relationships. *Will they be able to see me beyond my birthmark? Will they treat me differently because of it?*

Despite my expectations, I was one of the first of my girlfriends to have a boyfriend. I was always told that my birthmark was really cool. I honestly did not expect this reaction at all because I had feared judgment so much. But moments like that taught me that some people understand the desire to be seen and respected without being pitied. It was not the attention that helped me; it was the support the relationships offered while building my confidence. It made me realize my worth more than ever.

One of the most meaningful things a partner ever said to me was "It's just a part of you, as much as your hair or your eyes. I don't even notice it anymore; it's just you." That moment stayed with me because it made me realize that, sometimes, the fear of judgment is worse than reality.

One time, I met a guy at a birthday party. I was recovering from laser treatment, so I was wearing a lot of makeup that night. We talked a lot. No makeup is permanent, and it started rubbing off on my cheek. I didn't notice until I went to the bathroom. I felt a wave of embarrassment; he must have seen what was underneath my makeup and realized I was trying to hide something. When I returned, I decided to be upfront and told him the reason purple spots were showing through. I held my breath, waiting for his response.

He just shrugged and said he had noticed, but it didn't bother him. I was relieved. It showed me that it was okay to be different and that most people are able to see beyond looks. Character is worth more than looks could ever be.

## FINDING REPRESENTATION AND VISIBILITY

As I grew up, I rarely saw people with port-wine stains—neither in real life nor online. Whenever I do see someone in public, I get so excited, even though I never approach them. I should start doing that, actually.

Finding people with port-wine stains online is even harder. There are only a few influencers who have them. That's why I'm so grateful to be a part of this book. I want teenagers like me to be able to go online and find the information, support, and acknowledgment they need. Especially during adolescence, it is crucial to know that you're not alone. There are people like you out there, even if you haven't met them yet.

I hope people with visible differences never feel as if they have to hide or disregard their worth. My message is also directed to parents of children with visible differences; education and parenting are the keys to building your child's confidence.

And if you're a parent considering laser treatment for your child, please do it. Not because we want to hide our condition, but because growing the strength and confidence to embrace it is a long, challenging journey.

I challenge you to rethink beauty standards and what society perceives to be "normal." There is not just one way to think about beauty. It appears in all shapes and forms! I want to give a huge thank-you to the skin-difference community. Writing down my experience has made me realize just how far I've come. Everyone's journey with their birthmark is different because each one is unique—just like us! And that uniqueness is our Strength!

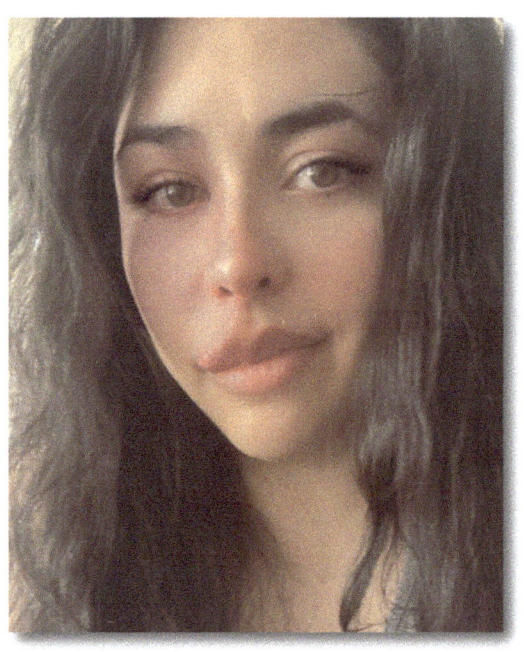

"With a vascular birthmark, there is often a misconception that it can simply be taken off as if it were some sort of sticker."

# THE JOURNEY
## *Hanna Prangner*

I still remember the day that I came home from school, ran to the bathroom, and sat on the counter. I grabbed a small comb, parted my hair on the right side, and watched as my hair fell over the left side of my face. I scrunched my legs up and zoomed in to look closer at myself in the mirror. This was the moment that I saw myself the way everyone else did.

I looked at my deep-purple port-wine stain on the left side of my face, smiled, and saw the purple pigmentation of my gums on the left and the pink gum on the right. I also saw the droopiness of the side of my lips. I looked down and could feel tears filling my eyes. My left eye got more red than it usually was as I cried. I mentally crawled into a hole—all of these feelings at the tender age of six.

As I recall this, I wish I could go back, open that door to the bathroom, where my younger self was sitting and feeling the bitter sting of insecurity, and just embrace myself in the warmest hug, knowing that everything would be okay.

My childhood was a little different than that of most kids. We lived in Texas, but my dad and I flew to San Diego, California, for my treatments. Because I was so young, they had to put me under full anesthesia for a ten-minute laser treatment. As I got older and could sit through it, the process changed. The nurse applied a thick layer of numbing cream and a cellophane wrap so that the cream would really numb the area. After about fifteen minutes, the cream was removed, and I was given numbing shots from the top of my eyebrow, down to my cheek, and inside my mouth. They put an eye shield over my left eye to protect it from the laser and prevent me from opening my eye. They covered my right eye with gauze and tape.

I could feel the laser at times; it felt as if a rubber band were being snapped against my skin. After every zap, they sprayed the affected area with a cooling mist. The pain was tolerable, but it was a type of pain I could never get used to. There was a smell of burning hair as the laser got near the hairline. The left side of my top lip was also lasered and even my gums to help with the purple pigmentation. After the laser treatment, my face was swollen. There were also purple pencil-eraser-size dots all over my face.

Then the recovery process began. I applied an absurd amount of ointment containing vitamins A and D and at times fell asleep with an ice pack on my face. I went through this every two to three months for years until I was in high school.

As a young girl, I attended a private school. The bullying of two girls began immediately and never ended; it was constant. Kids can be cruel, but so can adults. There was a teacher who, simply because I looked different, made the horrible assumption that I should be in a public school where special education was offered. I always felt the need to prove myself, and this feeling made me extremely quiet and shy.

Before meeting the cruelness of the world, my parents said that I was always a happy, playful kid. My mom wanted to help me as best she could, so she introduced me to the use of Dermablend foundation. Right when I thought I looked like everyone else, those two girls got a bucket of water and splashed me with it; they laughed hysterically as I ran to the bathroom and saw the smeared makeup washing away. I was desperate at this point to be left alone, but I also had the need to fit in.

The bullying got so bad that after five long years of silence, I finally broke down and told my parents what was happening at school. They immediately took me out of the private school and put me in a public one. This stage of my life was different; as a young girl, I was more aware of wanting to do my hair, to really get my makeup right, and to look a certain way to fit in. It was a struggle. I had extremely short hair, glasses, and braces.

It wasn't until high school that I discovered what I liked and developed some idea of what style was. I woke up at 6:30 a.m. and had to be at school at 8:00 a.m., but I still spent extra time doing my hair and makeup. However, for some people, I was always going to be the girl with the birthmark.

I developed a crush on a boy, and I remember sitting in class and writing a note to him. I folded it into a small square and drew a little heart next to my name. I stared at the clock, and the moment the bell rang, I rushed over to my friend and handed her the note that she was going to give to my crush. I remember being at my locker, and from across the hall, I watched as she walked over with a big smile and handed him the note. He opened it and looked over at me, but then he gave the note back to my friend who then turned around, her smile gone.

I asked her, "What did he say?" When she said nothing, I insisted on knowing. I told her that, whatever it was, I could handle it.

She turned to me and in a quiet voice said, "He said that you'd be pretty if you didn't have that thing on your face."

In my chest, I felt a deep sting that traveled slowly to the bottom of my stomach. It felt as if I had dry-swallowed a pill. The rest of the day felt like the slowest day ever. When I got home after school that day, I experienced a feeling of déjà vu as I stared at myself in the mirror, trying to figure out what I could do differently. I remember crying because I knew there was nothing I could do. I had exhausted all options.

The one thing I couldn't do at that stage in my life was accept myself in all ways. My mental health was a very serious struggle for me in high school. I was such a recluse I became almost mute. I never wanted to hang out with any of my friends and family or participate in any sort of activities. I was reminded, just by looking in the mirror, that I was not normal according to societal standards. The struggles to fit in seemed endless to me at that time.

Being a young teen, I had to focus on other health issues as well. Laser treatments were not as frequent, but the trips to my ophthalmologist were. Up until I was eighteen, I went to a pediatric eye doctor who specialized in glaucoma. I then transferred to a local doctor, and at times it was a roller coaster. Technically, a stable eye pressure is ten to twenty-one; with glaucoma, it still needs to be within that range, but it often exceeds twenty-one. When it does, there can be issues.

So what is glaucoma? Glaucoma is an eye disease that causes fluid buildup in the eye, which can damage the optic nerve. There aren't always symptoms. Some people say they experience headaches behind the eye, vision loss, or more floaters in their vision. There are many things now that can help keep the eye pressure at a healthy range. Eye drops and surgeries are usually the go-to treatments.

I am currently on three eye drops, and ever since I can remember, my eye has always been red—not necessarily because of the glaucoma, but because of the preservatives in the eye drops. I have gotten used to my eye looking more pink than it should and to people assuming twenty-four seven that I have severe allergies or even pink eye.

As you're reading this, you may ask, "Why don't you use redness-relief eye drops?" The answer? A lot of soothing agents and certain medications can raise my eye pressure, so I would rather not risk it.

I have had two trabeculoplasty procedures, which is laser in the eye to relieve the fluid buildup often seen with glaucoma. It helped for a while, but not the way the drops have. The procedure itself was more uncomfortable than painful. Laser treatments helped keep my pressure low for a while as well, but the importance of laser treatments is to help prevent issues such as the birthmark becoming more bumpy, which can lead to issues like itchiness and bleeding.

I mentioned my gum and lip being affected as well. Thankfully, my gums are fine, but aesthetically one side is purple, and the other side is light pink. My lips, however, are a different story. It was a little droopy on the left side. At a young age, this very much affected my self-esteem, and after visiting three different plastic surgeons, I found a doctor whom I was comfortable with when it came to performing a vermilionectomy. He surgically removed a total of eight millimeters of extra tissue on the left side of my lips. The recovery process was long, but worth it. I remember looking in the mirror, and my upper lip was swollen. I could see what looked like corset stitches. I got emotional because for the first time in my life, when I smiled, I actually truly looked as if I was smiling.

With a vascular birthmark, there is often a misconception that it can simply be taken off as if it were some sort of sticker. Finding the right dermatologist with the right laser is crucial.

I made the mistake of having laser treatments with a laser that barely penetrated the surface of my skin, and it caused a bad skin irritation.

On the other hand, having a tech who knows the settings is also just as important! I had an incident in which the laser setting was so high during one treatment that it actually looked as if a circular, pea-size chunk of skin had been burned off near the philtrum of my face. It hurt so bad. I had to wait for that to heal, and the solution was to fill it with collagen. It isn't as noticeable now, but it is a small scar. Unfortunately, these things can happen during treatments, but after that, it took me a while to ever want to attempt laser treatments again.

One day, my dermatologist told me, "Hanna, I think this is where we need to consider stopping treatments."

I remember standing up, looking in the mirror he had on the wall of the room, and saying, "My birthmark is still there."

He laughed and said, "It's never going to go away one hundred percent, but you have to find a point where you look at how far you have come and are happy with the results."

He was absolutely right. Having a skin difference made me realize just that. I remember the drive home—looking out the window and realizing that I had not been in the correct frame of mind while having my laser treatments. The whole time, I thought I was going to receive laser treatments until my birthmark was gone. Instead, I had to find a way to be okay with the fact that it would never go away. I was never going to just wake up one day and find that, suddenly, my birthmark and glaucoma were gone. Through self-reflection, I had to come to terms with the medical facts.

My birthmark has made me cry so much from sheer fear of being out of control. It has also allowed me to meet a part of me I didn't know existed. Today, I look back on many memories, and I need to acknowledge how much my parents fought for me to realize my own self-worth, especially when I was too young to see it. They never let the opinions of others cloud what they knew was best for me, as their daughter.

As a kid, I used to beg and plead to stop treatments. As an adult, I need to say thank you to them for not listening to me. Of course, I was afraid. And now, as a parent, I can't imagine seeing your child in that situation—numbing creams, anesthesia, bullying, and mental health battles. I hope whoever reads these stories knows that there's an entire community out there waiting to hear your story, so go and write it and let yourself be found.

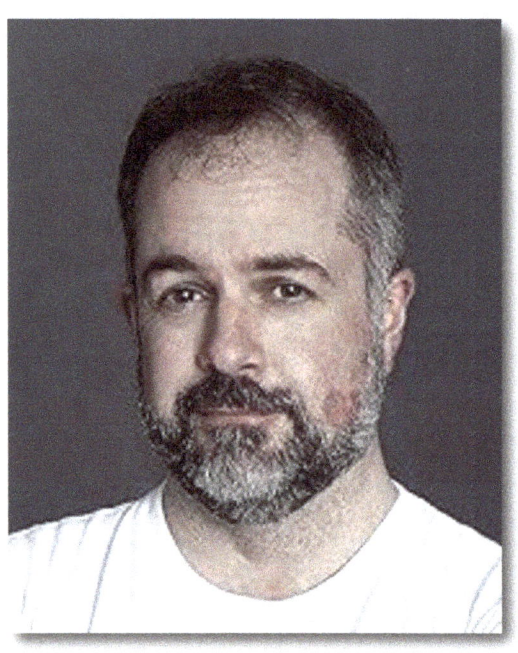

"Thinking that I was as much of an outlier as Joseph Merrick, the Elephant Man, I learned at an early age that people are outright assholes to anyone who is different. And children are the worst. The absolute worst."

# THE DAY I LEARNED MY NAME

*J. Brian*

There's always been some confusion about my name. When my parents got married, there were family members on both sides of the aisle with significant (generally unfounded) reservations. There were no objections on the big day, but few were overly excited about the match. Six months was the general consensus.

A few years later, when I came along, my folks attempted to mend fences. Long wanting a son named Brian, my mother conceded to James Brian in order to keep with my father's familial traditions. Privately, they both agreed that I would be called Brian, except in legal situations or when registering for anything…ever.

And so the confusion began.

Now, the nice folks over at Birthmark.org define a port-wine stain (PWS) as:

> …*a congenital, cutaneous vascular malformation. It involves post-capillary venules which produce a*

> *light pink to red to dark-red- violet discoloration of human skin....*
>
> *...PWS should not be considered a cosmetic problem but a disease with potentially devastating psychological and physical complications. Detailed studies have documented lower self-esteem and problems with interpersonal relations in PWS patients.*[1]

And that's important because on the left side of my face is what a child psychologist once described as "a fairly prominent birthmark." To give you a visual, imagine a painting of the Starship Enterprise being chased by the Hawaiian Islands, rendered entirely in bright red.

Now, as an adult, I intellectually understand that it's just a birthmark. I had the good fortune that there are no physical complications that accompany my birthmark, as that can be a sign of extremely serious underlying medical conditions. But I grew up in the 1980s and did not personally know anyone else who had a birthmark on their face. Well, I knew of one other person—Mikhail Gorbachev, premier of the USSR, colloquially known as the Evil Empire. There were no movie stars, no athletes, no musicians, no supermodels, and no other prominent popular-culture figures with a birthmark. I was the only one, the leader of the bad guys. Thinking that I was as much of an outlier as Joseph Merrick, the Elephant Man, I learned at an early age that people are outright assholes to anyone who is different. And children are the worst. The absolute worst.

This carries absolutely no legal weight, but if in your journey, you come across kids picking on a little kid with a

---

[1] The emphasis added is mine, and if I could emphasize it more, I would.

birthmark, you have my written permission to smack the little bullies around.[2] Even as an adult, I have no tolerance for bullies. Donald Trump mocking a disabled reporter told me all I needed to know about his character.

I digress. At one point, there was a kid who told me that my birthmark looked like the Starship Enterprise, as I mentioned earlier. He was, in fact, the first person to tell me that. The kid took a Rorschach test using my face and told me about it…to my face. And I realized it was quite possible, even quite probable, that everyone did that all the time…and would continue to do so for the rest of my life. No matter what my parents wanted to call me, I'll be forever known as the Kid with the Birthmark. I bet that'll be fun.

Now, when Irish eyes are smiling…they usually belong to someone who is up to something. And when I was a little boy, that aphorism definitely applied to me. When I was about the age of eight or maybe nine, my uncle, recognizing in his nephew a certain familial trait of smiling eyes, took me aside to explain some things to me. A few basic facts of life. Not the birds and the bees, but something much more consequential to a mischievous elementary-school-aged child.

Now, this was a man who grew up with a bright, flaming-red head of hair that, in his prime, was likely visible from space. His big sister, my mother, had christened him the Conover Street Comet, as he was always running up and down the streets, playing with the other children. From their apartment, he was easy to spot among his friends, a bright-red dot standing out among the other boys. And that's what he wanted to educate me about.

---

[2] Yeah, I know, that's a terrible attitude to have, but it's the one I've got.

He explained that standing out visually did not go hand in hand with getting away with things. When something happens—for example, when you're playing ball with your friends, and a window is broken, a car gets scratched, or fresh paint gets smeared, etc.—the adults will ask, "Who did this?" And even on the odd occasion when I wasn't the perpetrator, there was a good chance "That kid with the birthmark, he was there!" would likely be the reply.[3] "You may not get blamed, but they'll remember that you were there" was his advice to me. Again, that's my name—the Kid with the Birthmark.

I bear no specific ill will to any of the kids who picked on me because of the birthmark; they were kids. Obnoxious children—who generally didn't know better. Did I just describe most of the kids in history? Well, judging from who we've grown up to be, probably. But who knows what battles they were fighting in their own personal development. What bogeymen stalked their closets. Sometimes, though…sometimes…one person can completely alter your spin.

When I was a senior in high school, I worked after school at a law firm. It was a good gig, much cleaner and more prestigious than slinging burgers or pumping gas. I worked directly for the office manager; an amiable lady named Jane. My job was to take over errand-running and office-filing chores from the morning guy—a retiree named Dick—once I got out of school. It was a very professional environment and a worthwhile experience for a high school kid who was considering the legal profession.

When I got to work, my primary responsibility was to take care of any packages that needed to be delivered to the local corporations whose business was the lifeblood of the firm. So

---

[3] I assure you, this provides no legal protection, whatsoever.

I'd grab them and drive from office building to office building in Northern New Jersey, delivering leases, legal agreements, and I don't know what else. When that was done, I'd head back to our office where there would be a pile of case files that the attorneys had finished working on and needed to be refiled.

One day, after I'd been there for six months, a file in the "pile-o'-files," as we called it, had a Post-it note on it. It was a case file from the office of Mr. Bullwinkle, an attorney who I thought was a genuinely good guy. He was always friendly and said hello to the lowly office errand boy, asked me about college and life plans, and politely listened to whatever idiotic nonsense I was probably spouting in return. A nice guy. The Post-it read: "Katie—Have Dick, Jane, or Spot put this back in storage." Suddenly, I had been rechristened—no longer the Kid With the Birthmark, but now Spot. So I guess it turns out that grownups can be assholes too.

I was later to learn just how much worse they could be, but at sixteen, damn, this was hurtful. A grown man, fully realized in his adulthood, both personally and professionally, scoring some chuckle points with his eye-candy secretary at the expense of a pimply-faced high school kid. I'm sure he shared that around the office a few times. It's too perfect not to.

I kept the Post-it note as a reminder of what people who are nice to your face can actually be like behind your back. In college, a girlfriend who was bright beyond her years convinced me to throw it away, and physically I did. Mentally, though, the resentment lives rent-free right upstairs, matted and framed and featured prominently on the flypaper that is my mind.

I've wrestled with this particular resentment a lot. It is one of the few instances in which I have a hard time identifying my part in its genesis. Twenty dollars says that Mr. Bullwinkle doesn't remember me at all. The only reason it exists is because I keep it alive. It's been over twenty-five years.[4] I no longer bear the man ill will, and I wish I could forget the whole damn occurrence.

The problem is that, situationally as a joke, Dick/Jane/Spot… it is kind of funny. I recognize that. And it pisses me off on a lizard-brain level, which my higher level makes worse. Why does it make it worse? Because I think my resentment stems from the fact that I can see myself making the same type of joke… and I know that in the past, I have. And maybe what I really resent is that I have that capacity within myself. And so, thusly armed, I face the challenge of being a better person in the future.

And when we meet, you can call me Jay.

---

[4] LOL, well over twenty-five years…

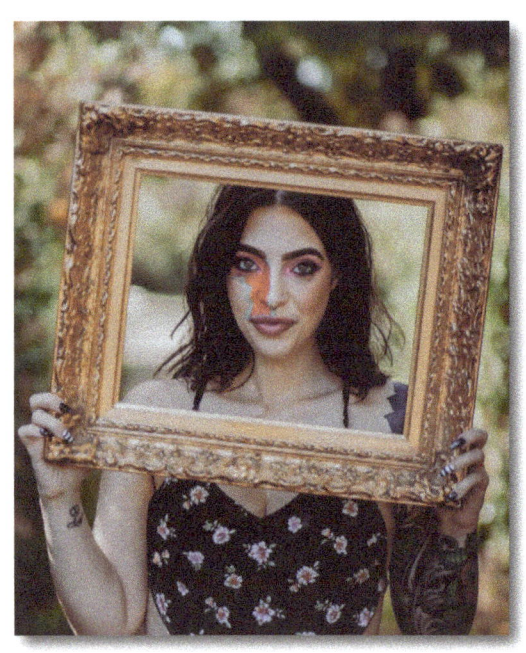

"I think about thirteen-year-old Jessica a lot. I talk to her all the time. I tell her how she's obviously gorgeous, barefaced and all."

# BIRTHMARKED BADASS
## MY STORY OF HEARTBREAK, SELF-LOVE, AND FORGIVENESS

*Jessica Weckherlin*

"You look like Two Face." It was the first time I remember realizing that I looked different. "You know, from *Batman*!" I was seven years old and in the second grade at Saint Maria Goretti Catholic School in Arlington, Texas. My classmates and I were having free time away from our desks. A little boy named Leonard came up to me, pointed at my face, and said the words that made my heart sink. I stared back at him, confused. I had never been called a name before, at least not to my face, not that I remembered.

Let's start from the beginning. To say my mom had a difficult birth experience would be an understatement. She was in labor for nineteen hours. My mom breathed and pushed, breathed and pushed, breathed and pushed. She breathed and pushed until she couldn't anymore. Rather than deciding to do a cesarean, the medical staff told her to breathe and push some more as they pushed down on her belly and instructed my dad to do the same, alongside them, with all his might as the doctor pulled me out with forceps.

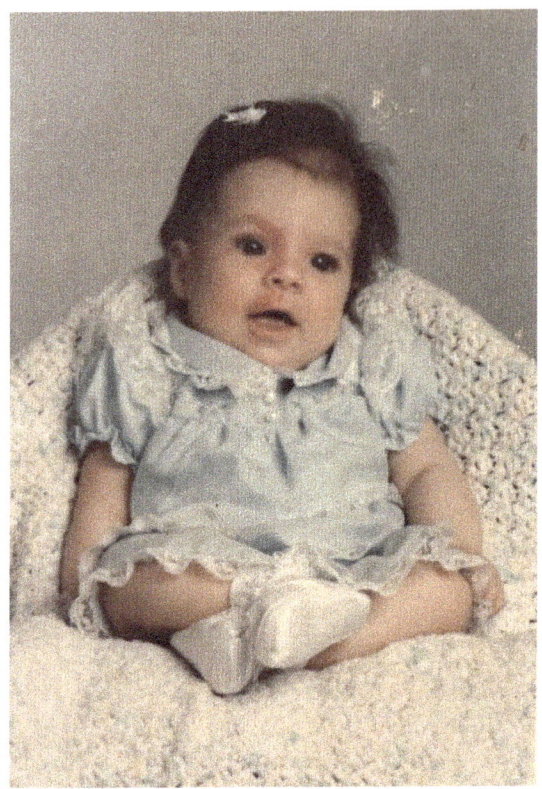

I was their first baby to make it earthside. I can't imagine my parents' anxiety and fear since this didn't seem to be going as planned. After a lot of frustration and tears, I came out screaming with a head full of thick, almost-black hair. I had ten fingers, ten toes, weighed in at eight pounds thirteen ounces, and had something peculiarly red on the right half of my face.

It was January 1987, before the days of Google. My parents immediately assumed the redness on my face was from the forceps, but my pediatrician, Dr. Rasmussen, told them it was a port-wine stain (PWS), which is a series of swollen blood vessels right under the skin. And that was it. No further explanation of PWS. Ever. The next day, my mom's ob-gyn told her they should have done a cesarean.

My parents are wonderful and did their best with the tools they had, which wasn't much. They shared stories with me about the many times strangers questioned them about my face when I was a baby. They said multiple people insinuated that I was abused and questioned them on how they cared for me. People would ask, "Was she burned?" or "Did she fall?" There just weren't a lot of resources, information, or representation at the time. My parents were on an island of their own. They didn't know anyone else with a PWS...until Dr. Rasmussen referred them to a friend who was doing pulsed-dye laser (PDL) treatments, which became the gold standard of treatment for PWS in the early 1980s.

PDL targets the hemoglobin within the blood vessels, causing them to fade and shrink. My parents started taking me for PDL treatments when I was about two years old. It was still new back then and had a long way to go. No, they weren't perfect.

My first treatment, the laser was turned up too high, and it burned me. That's why I have cratering on my nose. I didn't know until much later in life that I was born with a perfectly smooth nose. I always thought I was born with the texture I have, but my parents told me a few years ago that wasn't the case.

I was two years old and ready for another treatment. My parents wanted an early appointment to accommodate whatever else they had going on that day. My previous visits with this doctor were at the hospital, but this appointment was scheduled for the first time at her new stand-alone medical building.

It was 1989, so long before everyone carried cell phones, and one of my mom's coworkers called before we left for the appointment and said the doctor's office called her work line and canceled due to an emergency, never telling my parents the reason for the emergency. Later, the news reported that the little girl who had that early appointment had passed away.

They had their lines crossed on the oxygen tank and gave her too much gas. Her little body gave out, and she didn't wake up.

My parents were shaken to their core and spoke with the doctor after the incident, sharing their concerns. I had been getting treatments from that same doctor for about a year without any major life-threatening issues. The doctor told them that as a mother, she completely understood where they were coming from and assured them I was in good hands. After that incident, I went to just one more appointment before my parents decided to pump the brakes on treatments. I think they couldn't get over what happened to that little girl and decided it just wasn't worth it.

I think about that little girl a lot. I know nothing about her. I wonder what her name was. I wonder if she liked playing princess and with Barbies. I wonder what her birthmark was like. I wonder what she would be like today. Would we have crossed paths? Sometimes, I wonder, *Why her and not me?* This internal question has always caused deep introspection. My relationship with God has been a roller-coaster ride. I know things happen and people suffer for reasons we will never know. Sometimes, things simply remain unexplained.

All I know to do, now, as an adult who has gone on one hell of a healing journey, is to send that little girl all my love and gratitude. So to that little girl, "Thank you, thank you, thank you. We are doing some big work here earthside. Thank you for the work you did while you were here. Thank you for the joy you most certainly brought to the people whose lives you touched. Thank you for being an inspiration to me and for being with me on this journey. I promise I won't let you down."

Growing up with a visible difference is not for the faint of heart. My parents did an AMAZING job at making sure I felt loved, accepted, and for lack of a better word, normal, whatever that means. It wasn't until that day in the second grade, with Leonard, that I realized my birthmark was a "problem." What Leonard and I didn't know back then was he was mimicking what society had fed us as physically acceptable. Not to mention, kids are assholes.

Leonard had probably never seen anyone with a PWS. In his little boy brain, the only comparable reference was Two Face from *Batman* because my birthmark covers the right side of my face; my left side is completely untouched. In a way, I could see how a little boy may draw the line of comparison. However, I was a lot cuter than Tommy Lee Jones, thank you very much.

That moment was the beginning of me feeling "othered." It's as if something clicked in my brain and made me say to myself, *Oh, I don't fit in. I don't look like everyone else. I look like a villain. Does that make me…bad?* I didn't know how to process it. I don't even remember if I told my parents about it that day. Adolescence is hard enough for anyone, but for a kid with a visible difference, specifically on their face, I can tell you from personal experience it's a whole other level of difficulty.

From that day in second grade on, I vividly remember toeing the line between wanting to be seen and wanting to be invisible. I grew up as a dancer, so being seen onstage wasn't foreign to me. I loved performing. It was an outlet to express myself in ways I felt I couldn't offstage. What I didn't know then was that dance is one of the best ways to somatically process your emotions.

It all makes sense now, but I couldn't explain then why dancing not only felt good physically but felt good energetically. Not to mention the dopamine hit that happens when the spotlight hits you. It's so warm and blinding. You can't see the audience, but they can see you. It was a powerful tool to make people smile when inside I was feeling so much pain.

Sometimes, there was a lot of pain in being seen. I began to see people's micro-expressions when they first saw me. I noticed their quick double takes. I noticed when people stared, and as I made eye contact, they quickly turned their attention to something else. I noticed, when I met someone for the first time, how their eyes drifted to the right side of my face. I heard the whispers, specifically from other kids who asked their parents what was wrong with my face.

The older I got, the harder it was. Not only was I a tall, awkward, gangly pubescent girl with a PWS on half of my face, but I had a crooked smile and a gap between my two front teeth, which looked as if they had been parted by Moses himself. It was a rough phase. Naturally, I was boy crazy. I was just like any other girl whose room was basically a *Tiger Beat* magazine advertisement. Pictures of Jonathan Taylor Thomas and NSYNC adorned my walls from floor to ceiling. I daydreamed about what it would be like to have a boy interested in me the way I saw them pay attention to other girls at school.

One time, I had a HUGE crush on this supercute boy from another Catholic school at a speech and debate competition. I overheard him tell another boy I was a butterface. "She has a nice body…but her face…not so much." We weren't allowed to wear any makeup at school. Not even a little powder. My heart sank, but I wasn't surprised the supercute boy with the bleach-blond tips, conch-shell necklace, and popped collar on his Lacoste shirt didn't find me attractive.

The small, small world of Catholic school was a blessing and a curse. In a way, I felt safe because everyone knew everyone. Most of the kids had only ever attended that school, as I had, so at least I didn't find myself explaining my face to new kids every year. Each grade only had fifty kids, twenty-five in each homeroom, and I could probably count on one hand how many times, from first to eighth grade, we got a new student.

One of those students was a boy; let's call him James. I don't remember exactly when James came to Saint Maria Goretti, but we became close friends in the seventh grade. James was one of the few boys with whom I felt I could let my guard down. I remember him being funny, but not in a class-clown, show-off way. He was very kind and quiet. I never felt in danger with him. It never even crossed my mind that he would ever hurt me or take advantage of me in any way. I considered him my best guy friend. He was one of my only guy friends.

When we graduated eighth grade, we had a choice: go to the Catholic or the public high school. The decision was easy for me—public school, all the way. I was grateful for my time in private school, but I wanted more. I was ready to start over where no one knew me, and I wanted nothing more than to participate in the theater department.

My freshman year at the new school was a whirlwind. The school had 4,000 kids who all ate lunch at the same time. WILD. I settled in nicely. A couple of new friends took me under their wings and welcomed me into their group of friends. The best part? I was finally able to wear makeup. My experience with makeup up to that point was limited to dance recitals. My parents were really cool about allowing me to explore and figure out what worked best for me. With no support or resources, my mom took me to what felt like every single department store makeup counter available. I know drugstore brands have elevated their formulas recently, but in the early 2000s…oof. It was rough. Coverage? Don't know her! So from age thirteen, I had already invested in higher-end makeup to fit my needs. Even then, for high-end makeup counters, it was still rough. Makeup has come a long way since those days. I got the full coverage, all right, but the texture was cakey. I didn't care, though. New school. New look. New me.

I was on top of the world, until October 7, 2001, when I experienced one of the most heartbreaking betrayals of my life. I'll never forget it. I'm going to date myself here. I was at home on my family's computer, which had dial-up internet, using my FoxyRoxieHart13 AOL Instant Messenger and checking my Hotmail account. I received an email from James; we had kept in touch since our time at Catholic school and talked on the phone somewhat regularly. I told him how much I loved my new life at my new school. He, on the other hand, was struggling. I knew he missed me, and of course I missed him too. But we were thirteen years old. We were years away from being able to drive ourselves and had to rely on our parents for us to meet up.

The email was immediately weird. It was addressed to me, and only me, but it was as if he was talking to someone else. It went something like this: "I have this friend named Jessica. She's so beautiful." *Well, that's nice*, I thought to myself. I kept reading. The nice thoughts quickly subsided as I read the line: "I bought a knife, and I'm going to slit her throat open." My heart dropped. The email continued. He threatened another girl in our class and his mother. All of this was in great detail.

Trembling, I printed the email. My heart was racing. My hands were shaking. *What the hell? What does he mean?!* This was so out of character for that sweet boy I knew.

I ran upstairs to my room, shut the door, and called my best friend, Jackie. Jackie came to Saint Maria Goretti in the seventh grade. We instantly hit it off. She of course knew James from our SMG days, but also currently went to school with him at the Catholic high school. I read her the email because, you know, another thirteen-year-old would know what to do.

Jackie was beyond her years that night. She calmly told me to talk to my parents. That seems like the obvious choice now, but back then my head was spinning. She didn't freak out or raise her voice. She simply talked me off the ledge, calmed me down, and assured me everything would be okay. I went back downstairs and showed my parents the email. The cops were called, and my parents taught me an important lesson that night—grace.

School violence wasn't as rampant back then as it is now. My parents knew this kid. They knew this wasn't like him. Were they freaked out? Yes. Were they upset? Absolutely. My safety, and the safety of the others mentioned in the email, was of the utmost importance. They didn't press charges, though. More than anything, they wanted James to get mental health help.

The whole situation turned my life upside down. Not only was I the new girl, a very small fish in a gargantuan pond, hiding my visible difference to fit in, but now I was the new girl in the counselor's office, talking to security about my safety. I JUST WANTED TO BE NORMAL, FOR GOD'S SAKE!

I knew he was at a facility getting help, but then what? What if the mental health services he was receiving didn't work? What would happen if he tried entering the school to find me? These are thoughts I would never wish on anyone, especially a young kid at school. No child should ever have to worry about such things. Life never looked the same after that.

One thing that stayed the same: Jackie. She never left my side, even while going to separate high schools and eventually different states for college, and even different countries as we navigated our young adulthood. To this day, I consider that girl my soul sister. We have done every major life event together and have run into some intense challenges in our friendship.

My love and admiration for her has never wavered, though. It's an unbreakable bond. We always said that God made us friends because our parents wouldn't be able to handle us as sisters. We can't quit on each other now. We know too much about each other.

I did my best to conquer high school as normally as I possibly could. James doing what he did was a definite setback. It shaped me in ways I didn't fully process until I was an adult. You may be asking yourself what this has to do with my PWS. The answer for me is simple. Growing up and feeling as if the world were staring at you, and not for good reason, sucks. In my opinion, the least interesting thing about me is my PWS because I'm so much more than my visible difference.

With James, my PWS was a nonissue. It never came up in conversation. And although I was just a kid with no reference for what a "relationship" meant at that age—and dating wasn't ANYWHERE on my radar—James saw me. He truly saw me. He made me feel beautiful and confident, barefaced and all, in ways no boy ever had before. How could I go on and feel confident enough to be vulnerable and seen when my only experience with a boy ended with such trauma and chaos?

But I did date a couple of boys in high school. After what happened with James, though, combined with the inner struggle with Catholic guilt (if you know, you know), I kept my boyfriends at arm's length. I enjoyed being pursued, but I was a good girl, and good girls always stay in line. I never fully let my guard down.

As I got older and became more confident in who I was and developed my style through hair, makeup, fashion, and accessories, I subconsciously developed this mindset of "Oh yeah? If you're going to stare at me, I'll give you something to stare at!" I think I'm still a little bit like that today. I was exploring who

I was, and my parents really gave me space to express myself without freaking out about it. I wouldn't say this mindset was a bad thing, necessarily. However, it did create a vicious cycle of dressing and doing my makeup for the male gaze, and then becoming resentful when guys did pay attention because I would internally think to myself, *Dude, you have no idea what you're getting into with me. When you see me for who I really am, you're just gonna run like they all do. I'm too much, and painstakingly not enough.*

By no mistake, I ended up with a career in the beauty industry. I really wanted to be a dancer and actress. I auditioned for a performing arts school in New York City and was accepted, but even with financial aid, it was a stretch for my parents. I begrudgingly ended up going to the University of North Texas. I was happy to be there with some good theater friends from high school, but I was resentful I wasn't in New York.

College was not a good time for me. I didn't take care of myself at all. I didn't know a lot about depression at that time in my life. I was miserable and knew it wasn't the path for me. I was studying to be a theater and dance double major. They didn't offer the musical theater major when I was enrolled there. Just my luck.

I was in a costuming class, and I remember thinking to myself, *I think I like being behind the scenes more than I like being onstage, but how do I do this and actually make some money?* Capricorns, you know? Then it dawned on me. I was always the one French-braiding everyone's hair before dance recitals. I loved hair and makeup. I enrolled in beauty school and did the damn thing.

My career in the beauty industry has been extremely rewarding, but just like anything else, it has come with its hardships. My career is for another book at another time, but

I think part of what has made me so successful is I know to my core what it's like to look in the mirror and not love the face looking back at you. I know what it's like to cry out to the universe, "WHY ME? Why do I have this malformation? Life would be so much easier if I were just…pretty." But, oh my, I had so much to learn.

For being someone with so little confidence about how I looked while growing up, I had an insane amount of confidence in my abilities. If you weren't going to like me for my face, I'd make you fall in love with me for what I bring to the table with my value and my worth. I may be just a hairstylist from Arlington, but I have been on prestigious hair and makeup teams for New York Fashion Week and Nashville Fashion Week. I have done runway hair at Prince's old LA mansion and have participated in runway teams at hair shows with artists who have made such an impression on me personally and professionally. Maybe Mick Jagger was right: "We can't always get what we want; we get what we need."

When it comes to achieving your dreams, the how isn't always important. You simply follow the breadcrumbs and wait for the universe to show you. I didn't know how I was going to follow my dreams to New York and LA. I may have not fulfilled my dreams of being a dancer or an actress, but I still ended up in those spaces and doing what I love. The beauty industry is not what I wanted, but it's for damn sure what I needed. The universe had another plan for me. It's been incredibly healing for a girl like me—one with a visible difference—to touch the lives of everyone from a salon walk-in off the street to a celebrity. There's room for everyone at my table. We all deserve to feel beautiful.

Nothing has healed my PWS heart like the birth of my daughter. When I became pregnant, I felt all the roller coaster of emotions one normally does. I'm a little embarrassed to say it, but I will admit that my biggest fear was that she would be born with a PWS like mine. You must remember that I grew up with zero resources. In fact, even now as an adult, I get questioned by medical professionals all the time if I'm not wearing makeup.

It never dawned on me to Google "port-wine stain." Isn't that wild? It wasn't until much later in my adulthood that I started researching and learning about my own vascular malformation. A special friend in my life at the time encouraged me to look for a community on Instagram. So I did and started Googling. I had no idea PWS is not considered to be genetically inherited but is a sporadic gene mutation (the GNAQ gene) that develops two to eight weeks in utero. Remember my own birth story? My parents thought it was the result of birth trauma.

I will never forget being in labor and praying for my daughter's face to be clear. I didn't want her to have the life I have. I wasn't brave enough to voice this fear out loud, but, oh my God, I was praying HARD, "Please, God, please don't give my baby a port-wine stain." The moment I laid eyes on her, I couldn't believe it. What shocked me wasn't the fact that my prayer was answered, and she was PWS free; it was the realization that she was the most beautiful thing I've ever had the honor of seeing. It wouldn't have mattered if she had a PWS... or anything else, for that matter. It was like that scene in *The Grinch Who Stole Christmas* when his heart grew three sizes. Only mine grew a billion sizes. *Wow,* I thought to myself, *if this is how I feel about this tiny human I just met thirty seconds ago—she's the most overwhelmingly beautiful thing I've ever seen, and I don't think I've ever loved someone as much as I do at this very moment—that must be what my parents felt like when they saw me, the rainbow baby they prayed so hard for.*

It hit me like a bolt of lightning. We are worthy of love simply because we are. We are worthy of love because we exist. Not because of our clear complexions, hot bodies, or whatever the hell society has us brainwashed into believing makes us more valuable than the human standing next to us. I wish I could tell you I'm completely healed of my insecurities and have zero issues. I won't lie to you; they are still there. If it were up to me, I'd wear makeup every single day, but I'm raising a little girl now. I make a conscious effort to go makeup-free one to three days a week, depending on what we have going on. She needs to know her mama is confident and loves herself without the makeup. She needs to see the people do the double take, the stares, and the whispers when kids see me and point at me in the grocery store. I'm doing my best to show her beauty is in the eye of the beholder, even if it makes me want to jump out of my skin. She needs to know that humans are flawed, and that our flaws are our superpowers. She needs to know that if you're going to be anything, the most beautiful thing you can be is kind, and the most beautiful things you can do are give grace and have empathy.

I feel as if I began to master all this when I turned thirty. My daughter was about to be one year old just a few months later, and I knew I had so much to show and teach her. But, first, there was one thing heavy on my heart that I needed to let go. James. I thought about him every day, even more so after becoming a mother. I thought of what he did to me every time I looked at her, wondering what I would do if she somehow ended up in a similar situation. Did I have the grace in my heart that my parents did?

I looked him up on Facebook and found him. There he was, married and with a little girl of his own. I opened the Facebook messenger chat and sent him a short but sweet note. I told him I thought about him all the time, but that I was ready to let go of what happened all those years ago. I thanked him for truly seeing me when I felt so invisible, and I was ready to forgive him. I wished him happiness and asked him to honor that I wasn't interested in any sort of friendship. This was strictly a teary, cathartic goodbye.

He responded saying how much he appreciated my reaching out. He said he wanted to look me up and message me many times over the years but couldn't bring himself to do it out of fear that it wasn't appropriate. He thanked me for my forgiveness, but above all else, told me to thank my parents for giving him grace and making sure he got the help he needed. He was more than aware that if my parents had pressed charges, he would never have gotten the help he needed, and life would look a lot different.

I responded not with words, but with a heart. There were no words. Just a lot of love and peace for thirteen-year-old Jessica.

I think about thirteen-year-old Jessica a lot. I talk to her all the time. I tell her how she's obviously gorgeous, barefaced and all. I tell her that her beauty really shines through her softness and bravery, how she is equally human and divine. I tell her about all of our badass adventures and all the love we experience. I tell her how proud she would be to see us today.

Oh, sweet girl, you truly embody what it means to be beautiful, and you don't even have to try.

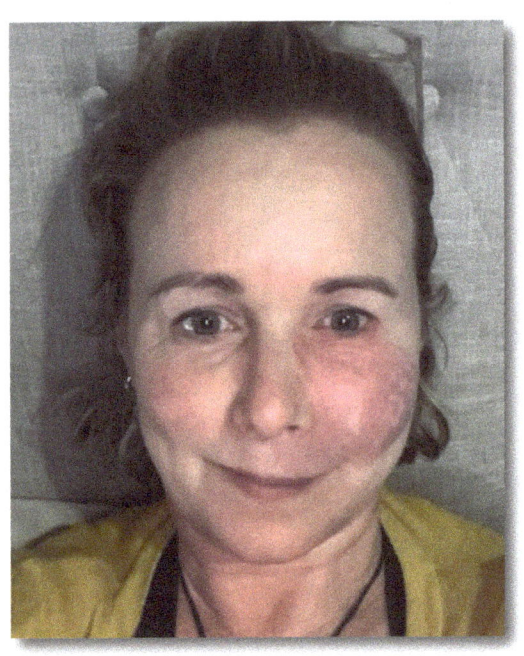

"I often wonder, do those who uttered the cursory words to me even remember them? Probably not."

# STICKS AND STONES
## *Kirsty Heather Ferguson*

I was born in the 1970s in Wellington, New Zealand. I went to a small inner-city school, and for the most part, my memories of those years were normal. I was simply me—Kirsty. Occasionally, new kids asked about my face, but since starting school at five years old, most people just accepted me as I was. I think our school was under fifty to sixty kids, so everyone knew everyone.

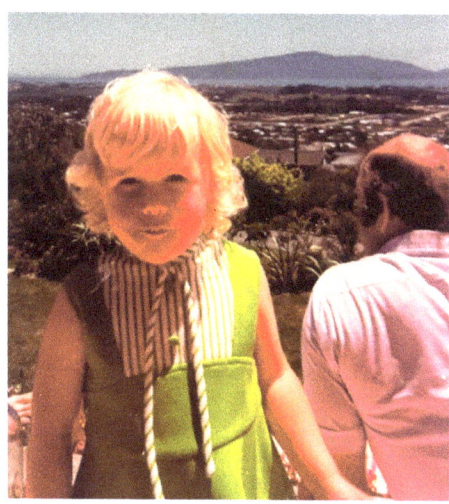

*Me in the 1970s on the Kāpiti Coast, New Zealand.*

## CHILDHOOD

My parents loved me for who I was, and from an early age, they put my facial differences into perspective. I have a PWS on the right-hand side of my face. It affects my teeth, gums, top lip, and eyesight. That eye was lazy; I had to wear glasses and a horrendous brown eye patch on top of them. I hated it. I ended up "losing" the patch and hiding it in the glove box of our car! Mum found it a few years later.

I have an older brother, born just a year before me, with congenital rubella. He is deaf, blind, and has what was then called brain damage—now referred to as cognitive delay. He requires twenty-four-hour care. My parents always reminded me that I was lucky that I could see, hear, talk, function, and make decisions. I was the sister who had to look out for him and be responsible. I knew nothing else.

My mum used to refer to my birthmark as my "bad side," telling me to turn a certain way for photos or to drape my hair just so. She never meant harm, but it took me until adulthood to rewrite that narrative in my head. Without realizing it, her words made me see my birthmark as something negative.

Growing up, I endured never-ending stares from strangers, probing questions from both adults and children, and cruel nicknames. Some even suggested I should feel lucky that everyone stared at me…because I was different. These were people who wanted to stand out, were punks, or liked attention.

Mum often said, "Sticks and stones may break your bones, but names will never hurt you," trying to help me cope with the unkindness. But as I reflect, I know that isn't true. Words hurt. Deeply. They made me self-conscious about my face and my appearance for most of my life.

I'm sure that people must have made hurtful comments to my parents as well. But they never shared those words with me. They simply accepted me. So did my grandparents, aunts, uncles, and their friends. No one in our close circle ever made me feel less than.

## PRIVATE SCHOOL

When I turned twelve, my parents decided that a private school would be a better option. They thought that with fewer students, there might be fewer stares and less cruelty. But even in that environment, I was not spared.

I still remember the classroom where the two girls who tormented me sat. I was next door. Their names were Emma and Alyshia. One knew my family; the other did not. Yet both called me "nappy rash face" and "beetroot face." Their pointing fingers, their cackling laughter, and their tears of amusement still echo in my memory. The pain they inflicted lingers, as raw today as it was then. I avoid college reunions and catch-ups because the thought of seeing them again fills me with dread.

I told my parents, and Mum made a phone call to confront Emma's parents. Emma, of course, denied everything at first. But after a few hours, the truth surfaced. Another call was made, and an apology followed—though I don't recall it. What I do remember is the sting of their words and the lasting impact they had on my mind and my self-esteem for all of my life.

I can only imagine what it must be like today for those with a PWS, with the internet and online trolling. If the words from my childhood can still bring me to tears forty years later, how much deeper must the wounds of online cruelty be?

The teenage years were already difficult enough back then. Today, they are so much harder. My self-esteem suffered. It impacted my choices, my friendships, and my confidence in ways I didn't even realize at the time. But the friends I have love me for me, they get me, and they are my biggest supporters.

## LASER SURGERY AND MAKEUP

Sometime around the age of twelve, I traveled to Sydney to see my aunt and uncle. On a visit to a mall, we heard an advertisement for Coverblend makeup. So I tried some, and the person mentioned a doctor in Sydney who used a laser on birthmarks. An argon laser. That trip, I came home with makeup. Later, I completed twelve hours (over a week, three sessions of four hours each, with a day's break in between) of laser treatments. Dr. Adriana Schibner was the doctor, and over the next five to six years, I had laser on my face, which, despite being grueling and leaving me unwell for the rest of the day, did lessen the purple color and size of the PWS on my face.

Laser treatments were tough, as I seemed to be allergic to every anesthetic they gave me to numb the pain. Each visit, I endured four hours of laser, left, and winced in pain for the next twenty-four hours while my skin swelled, blistered, and seeped what I can only assume was pus. It was quite an ordeal, very painful, and would often result in my throwing up.

By the time I left Sydney to return to New Zealand, I looked as if I had been beaten up and burned. Over the next ten days, my skin healed, peeled to almost-normal skin again, and then faded in color. I was lucky I never scarred. The doctor was very careful with the heat, as I had begged her not to disfigure me. However, the trips to Sydney stopped abruptly when Dr. Schibner became addicted to drugs and was sent to prison.

I was a bit young to remember much, but that was the end of laser for a while.

These trips altered my life in two ways. They introduced me to the world of makeup, which I still rely on today, even though I jumped into a world of lasers in the hope that one day my skin would be normal.

But through all of this—the stares, the whispers, the cruel words—I have learned to embrace who I am. My journey was difficult, but it shaped me into the person I am today.

Luckily, in 1998, I came upon a surgeon in New Zealand, in my hometown, who literally had an office just a three-minute drive from my house. When I was pregnant with my first child, Ally, a growth appeared, about the size of a raisin, on the edge of my lower eye. He swiftly removed it and encouraged me to come back for treatment. He is a kind and gentle man who zaps away swiftly and then sends you on your way. He has done a lot of research around birthmarks and their connection to cancer and is heavily involved in research to find a cure for cancer.

## ADVICE FOR TODAY

If I had any advice for parents, it would be to be your child's biggest advocate. Cheer them on, but understand that the words and actions of others are hard to handle, no matter what. They cut deep, and they ruin a person's self-worth. Therapy and coaching are excellent tools to build resilience, work through the damage, and allow grief to be unleashed. They are things I wish I had had access to way earlier in life, but that I have used both in adulthood. Someone recently said, as I cried after hearing more cruel words, "Why are you letting them still control you? Let go."

Keep your kids safe on devices and have a safety plan against cruel messages and online bullying. It is bad for teenagers with no facial issues, let alone those with differences. The messages can very quickly become toxic, too much, and cannot be erased. PTSD is real and alive. Screenshots are now evidence... It's so challenging out there.

Support your kids. Those who are cruel and have no heart will not stay friends for long. But be wary; this can take a significant toll.

For those with PWS who are the targets of cruel looks or words, had I been reliving these things today, I probably would have gotten way angrier! I often wonder, do those who uttered the cursory words to me even remember them? Probably not.

## PORT-WINE STAIN COMMUNITY

In the past year, I discovered and joined the PWS community through Instagram, after having first come across Paige Lauren Billot. For a long time, I watched her from afar, in awe of her bravery, and admired her tenacity and courage. What an awesome ambassador for anyone and everyone with a facial deformity or port-wine stain.

After watching many videos, I realized there was a lot to learn. I joined the community and started to make connections with people like me. This past year, I have learned so much about vascular birthmarks; it has been a real eye-opener. I am so grateful. I have had several Zoom calls and have exchanged many messages with other people with birthmarks around the world.

The first Zoom meeting, it was quite overwhelming to see so many people like me. It brought me to tears. It allowed me to find my people. My heart was filled. So thank you, internet, for bringing people together to feel a sense of connection, a community that actually gets it! One day, I hope to meet some of the many faces and connect in person. I will be so grateful for their acceptance, their understanding, and their aroha (love).

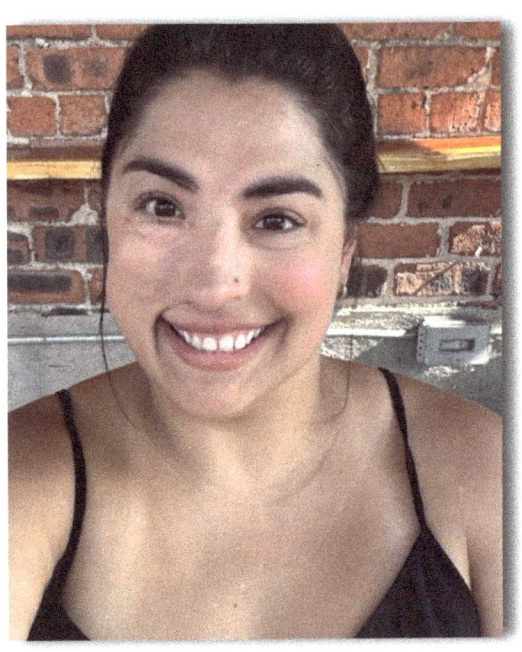

"So I sit here, on this crisp day in New York City, feeling the sun on my face and the weight of my past no longer holding me down."

# HOW I STOPPED LETTING MY BIRTHMARK DEFINE ME

*Lorena Bryant Hixson*

I sit at a picnic table in Riverside Park, overlooking the Hudson River and the New Jersey skyline. The crisp air brushes against my face, the sun warming my skin as I take in the city that once felt like an impossible dream. I look around and think about how far I've come, how I never thought I'd be here—here in this moment, in this city, in this life I have built for myself. It's easy to forget where I started, to lose sight of the battles I fought to get here. But, today, I remember.

I entered the world like any other newborn—tiny and full of possibility. But my journey took an unexpected turn just ten days later when a tiny red dot appeared on the right side of my face. What my parents initially dismissed as a harmless birthmark soon became a parent's worst nightmare. Day by day, they watched helplessly as this small mark grew with alarming speed, eventually engulfing the entire right side of my face.

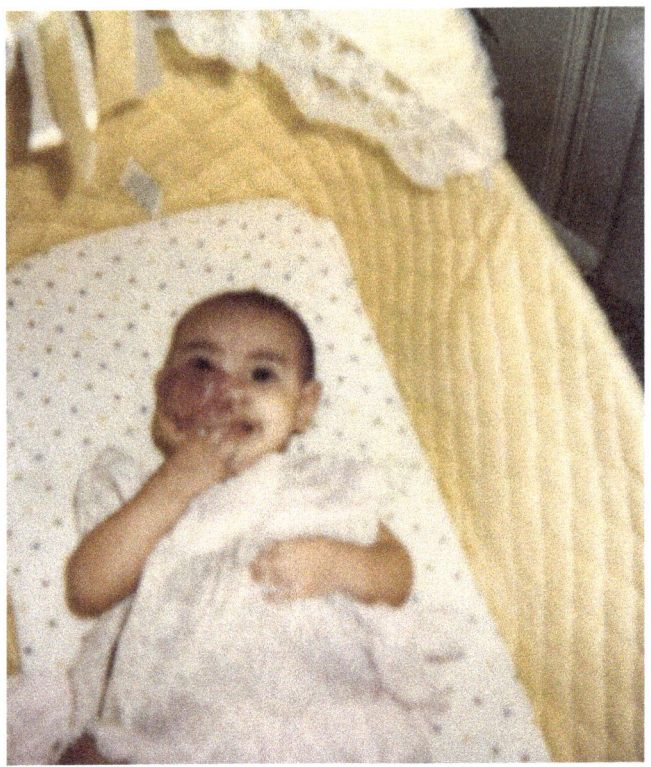

At three months old, my condition became life-threatening. Since no one could figure out what was happening, there was genuine fear that I might not survive or that I would live with severe cognitive deficits. Finally, a doctor in a neighboring city recognized my condition and connected my family with a specialist. That's when I was diagnosed with a cavernous hemangioma—a benign tumor that was both superficial and deep in the tissue. It was red, large, and ulcerated, growing aggressively.

Most hemangiomas shrink over time and don't require treatment. But mine was different. I had compromised vision and feeding, bleeding, airway concerns, and a high risk of permanent scarring. The situation was urgent. My case was sent to a specialist, in Florida, who insisted I needed immediate surgery.

Within forty-eight hours, my parents packed up everything, and we were on our way.

At three months old, I had my first surgery. It was a laser treatment to stop the tumor's growth. But that was just the beginning. What followed was a relentless cycle of surgeries every year until I turned twenty-one.

After my first surgery in Florida, my case was managed by a plastic surgeon in my hometown. Once the tumor stopped growing aggressively, the new focus became removing the remaining mass before it could cause further complications. But because the tumor was so large, they couldn't remove it all at once; doing so would have left a sizable hole in my face. Instead, they had to remove it in sections.

When I was in kindergarten, they implanted a tissue expander in my face—the same type of implant used in breast augmentation. The implant was inserted in the right lower side of my face where there was no damaged skin. The goal was to stretch the undamaged skin so when the bulk of the tumor was removed, this stretched skin could be used to replace the damaged skin.

By the time I was in middle school, surgeries had become second nature. The hospital was almost like a second home. My peers spent summers going on vacations or to camps. I spent mine under surgical lights, waking up to the familiar sounds of beeping machines and the post-op haze of anesthesia.

The process was exhausting, but in some ways, the hospital was one of the only places I felt safe. The nurses were kind. The doctors treated me with care. And for a brief moment, I wasn't just the girl with the tumor; I was a patient, someone they were helping.

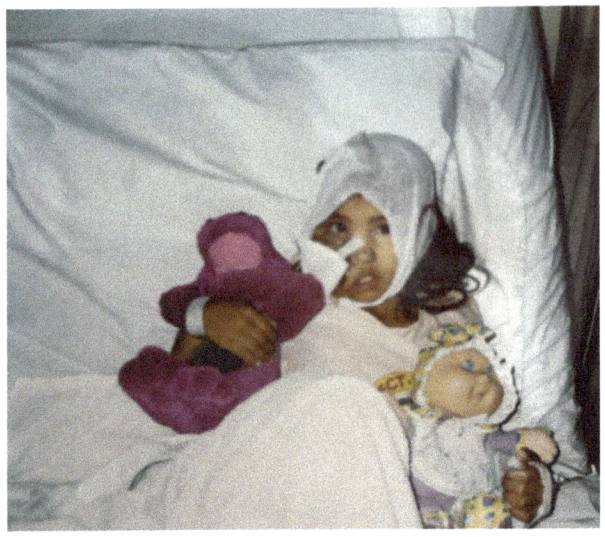

Being at the hospital was one of the only places I felt I truly belonged. I was surrounded by other kids who also had visible differences and scars, kids who understood the struggles I faced. I loved hanging out with the other kids; it was one of the few times I didn't feel the need to hide or cover up. I could just be me.

As I grew older, the surgeries became more focused on repair and reconstruction rather than tumor removal. Because the tumor had been so aggressive, it left significant scarring and skin damage. My plastic surgeon had to be strategic—rebuilding my face while making sure the skin remained functional and natural looking.

Even though my surgeries were life-changing, they weren't without complications. There were times when the healing process was slow, when procedures didn't go exactly as planned, or when I had to endure more pain than expected. But I never had the luxury of avoiding them. If I wanted to regain function and reduce the risk of long-term damage, I had to keep going.

The surgeries left scars, both visible and invisible. But I never truly saw those scars as a testament to my strength.

I saw them as marks of shame—reminders of what made me different, what made me feel as if I didn't belong.

When I was younger, the reflection I saw in the mirror didn't make sense to me. I didn't see a version of myself that felt worthy of love or acceptance. I felt like an outsider from a very young age. I remember the whispers, the stares, and the questions that followed me wherever I went. "What happened to your face?" people would ask, often in a tone that left me feeling like an outcast. The weight of those questions, the burden of people's unasked curiosities, was something I carried for years.

There's an immense pressure to fit in, to look like everyone else, to be what others think you should be. Growing up, I didn't have the understanding to process what was happening. All I knew was that I wanted to be seen for who I was, not for the marks on my skin. But even as I tried to hide, to camouflage myself in a version of me that the world would find more acceptable, I was always reminded that I couldn't outrun the truth of my scars.

So I did what I could—I hid. I lived a life that revolved around people-pleasing and avoiding conflict. I became adept at seeking validation from the outside, thinking that if I could just make people happy or look a certain way, I could somehow become worthy of their approval. But no amount of praise, no amount of attention, ever made me feel as if I was enough. It was never going to be enough because I wasn't giving myself the same love I was so desperately seeking from others.

For years, I lived in the shadows of my insecurities, constantly worrying about what others thought of me. I thought that by shrinking myself, I could avoid rejection or judgment. But the truth was, I wasn't avoiding anything. I was just making my life smaller and smaller until I could barely recognize myself. I had to be willing to stand in my truth, even when it felt as if the world might push me back down.

But, today, I know better. Running from the truth used to feel safe. But now I know the truth will always find you. And avoiding it is so much more painful than facing it head-on. I know that I am enough exactly as I am. And my scars? They are my story. When I stopped trying to hide them, when I stopped shying away from the very thing that made me different, I began to reclaim my power. My scars are not something to hide from or be ashamed of. They are the proof of my survival, my resilience, my strength.

But more than that, I want to share what I've learned—the deeper lesson beneath it all. It wasn't easy to get to this place. I had to make the decision to stop seeking validation from outside sources. I had to let go of the fear that everyone would abandon me if I spoke my truth. The more I leaned into the discomfort, the more I realized that the things I was most afraid of weren't nearly as powerful as the strength I was discovering within myself.

The most challenging part of this journey has been the process of unlearning everything I thought I knew about myself. It's been about reprogramming years of people-pleasing behavior, of doubting myself, of living in a world that constantly told me I wasn't enough. And, even now, there are moments I struggle to trust that I am enough without external validation, without the approval of others.

I want to keep healing, keep growing, keep being present. Because this life I am living now, it's better than anything I could have ever imagined. And the woman I am becoming, she is worth every ounce of struggle, every tear, every painful lesson.

When we speak our truth, we help others feel seen. We remind them they are not alone. And in doing so, we find the courage to stand tall, to claim our space in the world, and to embrace all the parts of ourselves that we once thought we had to hide.

If I could go back and tell my younger self anything, it would be this: life is going to be hard. There will be moments when you feel as if you can't keep going, when the weight of everything feels unbearable. But, one day, you will look around and understand why it all happened. Every painful moment, every heartbreak, every surgery, every time you felt as if you didn't belong—it was all leading you to this moment. To the realization that life isn't about chasing perfection or external validation. It's about unlearning the lies we've been told about who we should be and finding our way back to who we truly are.

So I sit here, on this crisp day in New York City, feeling the sun on my face and the weight of my past no longer holding me down. There was a time when New York City felt like a far-off fantasy, something I admired from a distance but never thought I could ever truly be a part of. A girl from small-town Tennessee, raised in the shadow of expectations, living a life shaped by constant self-doubt.

The woman I am today would have seemed unrecognizable to the girl I used to be. I've changed. My journey has been long, full of twists and turns, but it's also been incredibly worth it. It took me thirty-six years to find her, and I will never lose her again. For the first time, I feel as if I am truly living my dream. Not because I have everything figured out, but because I am present. Because I am finally in a place where I can embrace the unknown instead of fearing it. There is so much more I want to experience, so much love to give and receive, and I am grateful to be here for all of it.

I am becoming her—the woman I always dreamed of being. The fearless, strong, empathetic, confident woman I saw in my mind but never truly believed I could be. I still have fears. I still have moments of doubt. But I also know I am capable of more. I trust now that everything I want will come in its own time. The journey itself, with all its painful lessons, is where I am shaped into the person I am meant to be.

And for the first time in my life, I am not afraid of what's next.

Because I know now…I was always enough. And I always will be.

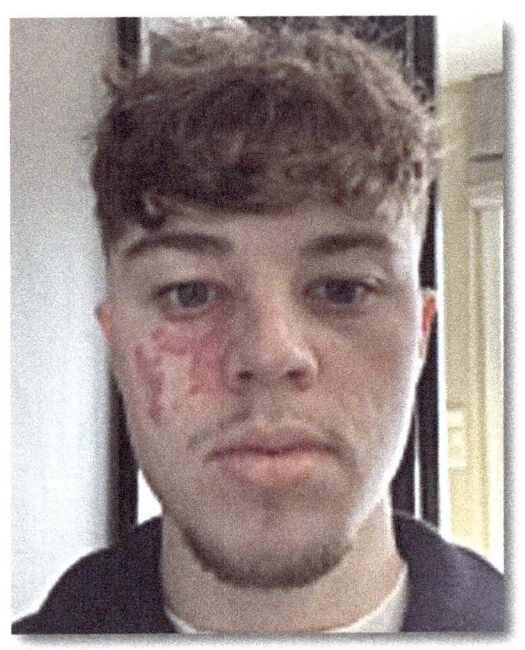

"It's not about hiding who we are; it's about having control over how we present ourselves to the world."

# MY STORY: BEYOND THE STARES

*Matthias De Potter*

### MY JOURNEY WITH A PORT-WINE STAIN

I was born with a port-wine stain covering the right side of my face. A deep-red mark—unmistakable, impossible to ignore. From the moment I came into the world, it was the first thing people noticed—long before they got to know me. As a child, I sometimes wished I would wake up and it would be gone. I'd stare in the mirror, rubbing at it, half-hoping it would just disappear under my fingertips. *Why me?* I would think. *Why this?*

### NO MIRACLE TREATMENTS

When I was little, my parents did what any loving parents would: they searched for a solution. Doctors recommended laser treatments—fifteen in total. The first ten were under full anesthesia. I was too young to remember most of them, but I do remember waking up with my face swollen and burning.

They promised the treatments would help. And in some ways, they did, but not in the way I had hoped. My birthmark became slightly lighter, but it never truly faded. When I didn't undergo treatments consistently, the redness always returned.

After a break, I decided to try laser treatments again when I was sixteen years old. This time, there was no anesthesia. I was fully awake, lying on a firm treatment table while the laser burned into my skin. It felt as if hundreds of needles were stabbing me over and over. My knuckles turned white as I gripped the edges of the table; my muscles tensed with each pulse of the laser.

I kept hoping that maybe this round would be different; after all that pain, all those appointments, I would finally see a change. But in the mirror, I still saw the same birthmark staring back at me. But at least, as a kid, there was one bright side. After every treatment, I got to pick out a present at the toy shop. I would walk in, cheeks still burning, knowing I had earned whatever I wanted that day. It was my only reward for enduring something that felt like punishment.

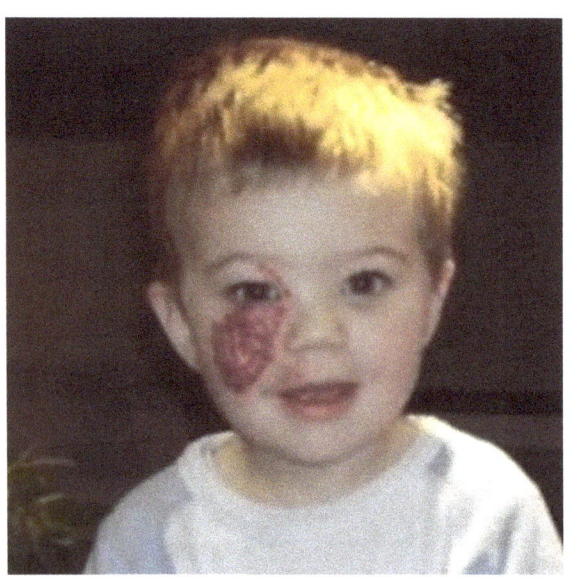

## THE UNEXPECTED TRAUMA OF THE HOSPITAL

Some of my most terrifying experiences weren't just about the pain of the treatments themselves; they came from the things I never saw coming. One time, after waking up from anesthesia, my vision was blurry, and I could only see out of one eye. But in my groggy state, I didn't really process it.

Then my mom started panicking. I could hear the fear in her voice as she grabbed my hand. "His eye is black!" she cried out. "He lost his eye!"

That's when the panic hit me. My heart pounded. *Have I really…? Is something wrong with my eye?* It turned out the surgeon had forgotten to remove the eye protection they used during the laser treatment. After some time, the surgeon came back and casually took it out, acting as if it was nothing—no permanent damage, no real injury. But that fear in that moment is something I'll never forget.

And then there was the other anesthesia incident. Apparently, I don't go under easily. One time, half under sedation, my body instinctively fought against it. I don't remember anything, but I've been told that three nurses had to hold me down to keep me on the table because I wanted to escape.

## THE REALITY OF GROWING UP DIFFERENT

If you've never had something that makes you stand out —something that always draws attention—you might not understand what it feels like to constantly be the center of unwanted attention. I wasn't just another kid at school; I was the kid with the red mark. The stares came first, then the questions. "What happened to your face?" "Did you get burned?" "Can you wipe it off?" Some were curious, some cruel. At school, some kids treated me as if I was some kind of joke, an easy target. There were days I was bullied from morning until the last bell rang—no break, no escape.

Football, something I loved, became another battlefield. I remember standing on the pitch, just wanting to play, and hearing kids on the sidelines yelling, "Maybe his birthmark gives him extra speed!" or "Don't get too close; it might spread!" The coach never stepped in. The other kids laughed. I stood there, fists clenched, pretending it didn't bother me. But it did.

Although, the worst part for me wasn't just the looks or rude comments; it was having to explain myself every single day, answering the same questions over and over again.

## THE FIRST TIME I HID MY BIRTHMARK

I still remember it vividly, the first time I covered my birthmark. Unlike what most people might think, it didn't happen in my bathroom with my mom's makeup. It happened in the hospital, where they have a department to cover skin conditions. A doctor applied camouflage makeup on my skin, blending and layering until, for the first time, my birthmark was as good as gone. I stared at my reflection, and for a moment, I couldn't believe what I was seeing. For as long as I could remember, my birthmark had been the first thing people noticed about me—the first thing I noticed about myself. And now it was just…gone.

A wave of relief washed over me. It was as if I had been carrying an invisible weight my entire life, and suddenly it was lifted. No more stares. No more questions. No more explaining myself to every person I met. For the first time, I felt what it was like to blend in, to just be.

But that relief was short-lived. It didn't take long for me to realize that the products available for people like me weren't made for real life. The makeup felt heavy on my skin, thick and cakey. It cracked after a few hours, settling into every fine line. It took ages to apply, layering and blending, only for it to rub off too easily. And worst of all, it wasn't designed to be good for the skin—it dried it out, clogged my pores, and made it more irritated over time. I had solved one problem, only to be met with another. If my birthmark had made me stand out, then wearing makeup made me stand out in a different way. A boy covering his face with makeup wasn't exactly normal.

Still, I kept going. Over the past ten years, I have tested every product I could find—high-end brands, professional camouflage makeup, and even custom blends. Yet nothing has truly met my needs. And I know I am not alone. People with skin conditions like mine deserve makeup that works for them, not products that force them to compromise between coverage, comfort, and skin health.

That's why I am changing this. I am developing my own medical-grade cosmetics—products specifically designed for people with skin conditions. Not just makeup that covers, but products that care. Products that are long-lasting, breathable, and won't feel like a mask. Makeup that doesn't just sit on the skin but actively nourishes and protects it.

That's how the idea for my own camouflage-cosmetics brand was born—not just to cover, but to care. To give people a choice. Because it's not about hiding who we are; it's about having control over how we present ourselves to the world. Because I know exactly what it's like to search for something better. And now I'm creating it myself. A community that sees me.

One of the most powerful moments in my journey wasn't about the product itself; it was about the people. When I shared my story online, I didn't expect the response I got. So many people—people with birthmarks, vitiligo, rosacea—messaged me, thanking me for putting into words what they had felt their entire lives.

I remember a teenager, from Morocco, who told me he had been denied jobs and couldn't find love because of his birthmark. He had been told, outright, that his birthmark was the problem. It was heartbreaking…and deeply unfair.

For some, love is harder; for me, it was a pleasant surprise. For years, I never let anyone see me without my camouflage. Not friends, not strangers—no one. And when I started dating my girlfriend, I kept up the routine. Each morning, I'd wake up before her, quietly slip into the bathroom, and apply my makeup so she wouldn't see me barefaced. I told myself it was better this way. That it would spare me the awkward conversations, the explanations.

But I couldn't keep it up forever. The day she finally saw me without it, I braced myself for…something. Shock, curiosity, maybe even hesitation. But she looked at me the same way she always had. It was just me. No judgment, no questions—just acceptance.

## REDEFINING BEAUTY THROUGH INNOVATION

I still wear makeup. Not every day, not because I have to, but because I choose to. And that's exactly what I want to offer others—the freedom to choose. For years, I searched for a product that truly worked for people like me. Something lightweight yet effective, something that covers time-efficiently, doesn't feel heavy, or harm the skin. But it didn't exist. So I decided to create it. This isn't just makeup; it's medical-grade cosmetics designed for real life. A product that doesn't just conceal, but cares. That lasts, breathes, and nourishes the skin instead of making it worse. Because no one should have to choose between confidence and skin health. I know what it's like to feel like there are no good options. And now, I'm creating one.

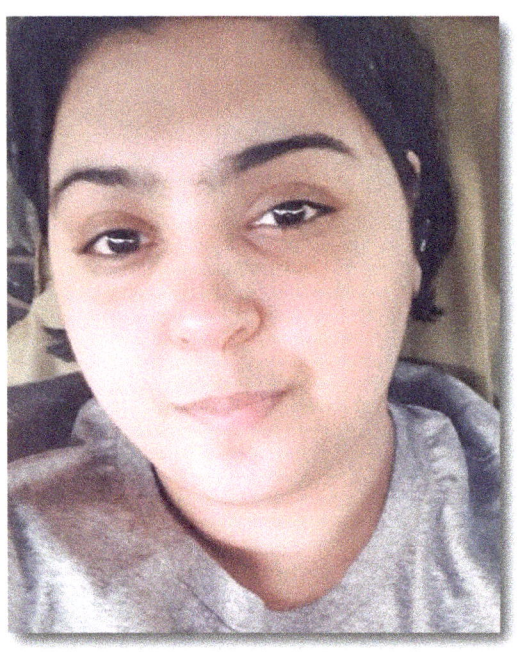

"I love when people ask me about my condition and my journey. It feels as if I did something great with my life, and I always thank God for everything that happens on my journey."

# MY STORY, MY JOURNEY
## Omaima Aladwani

My journey begins at eight years old with arteriovenous malformation (AVM). I was officially diagnosed two years later, at age ten. They said that there were no treatments; my only option was surgery in the USA. So in 2012, I went to Denver, Colorado, for the surgery, but it was not surgery; it was treatments. I had a lot of treatments in Colorado during 2012, 2013, 2015, and 2016.

I was bullied at school by girls more than boys. At age seventeen, in 2014, I started to share awareness in my community with friends and family.

At age ten, I was told that my AVM was present at birth, but it demonstrated at age eight. In 2013, I developed foot drop from the treatments in Colorado at age sixteen, but now I walk with a cane after I did physical therapy. They told me that my AVM is really big, deep, and hard at the same time.

I had a lot of treatments in Colorado between the ages of fifteen and nineteen. I started to look on social media for people who have AVM like me, and I found a lot of support groups and people who shared their AVM stories. I shared my story too. In 2020, I found other amazing groups of people with vascular birthmarks and met such lovely people. In 2021, I started to share my awareness on social media and found a lot of support. AVM has taught me to be who I am, to be humble, and not to stop sharing awareness. My story has helped a lot of people who have AVM. I'm always getting messages about it.

I had a lot of alcohol-injection treatments. In 2013, the doctor injected by mistake the nerve of my leg instead of the vein, and it's been one year of challenges with foot drop and a year of physical therapy and depression because of the bullies.

In Colorado, I met a wonderful friend who has helped me so much throughout my journey. She understands my condition, and she has supported me and become my best friend. I am really proud that I started to share awareness in Arabic and English; that helps me to find people globally, which makes me really happy and proud.

I am really grateful that I have a wonderful family—my mum and my lovely sister, Nour—who have supported me since day one. I am really blessed to have them in my life.

When I remember everything that happened on my journey, I feel so blessed and proud. I love when people ask me about my condition and my journey. It feels as if I did something great with my life, and I always thank God for everything that happens on my journey with AVM, during the treatments, surgeries, and experiences with foot drop and my disability.

As always, when I look back, I am so proud of myself. There is a quote I always repeat to myself; it has made me a strong woman.

> *Always do anything that you feel good about. Anything your mind says, do it. Don't care about the bad things that people say. Just be yourself. That will make you strong, humble, proud, and*

*blessed. At the same time, always feel blessed for what you have.*

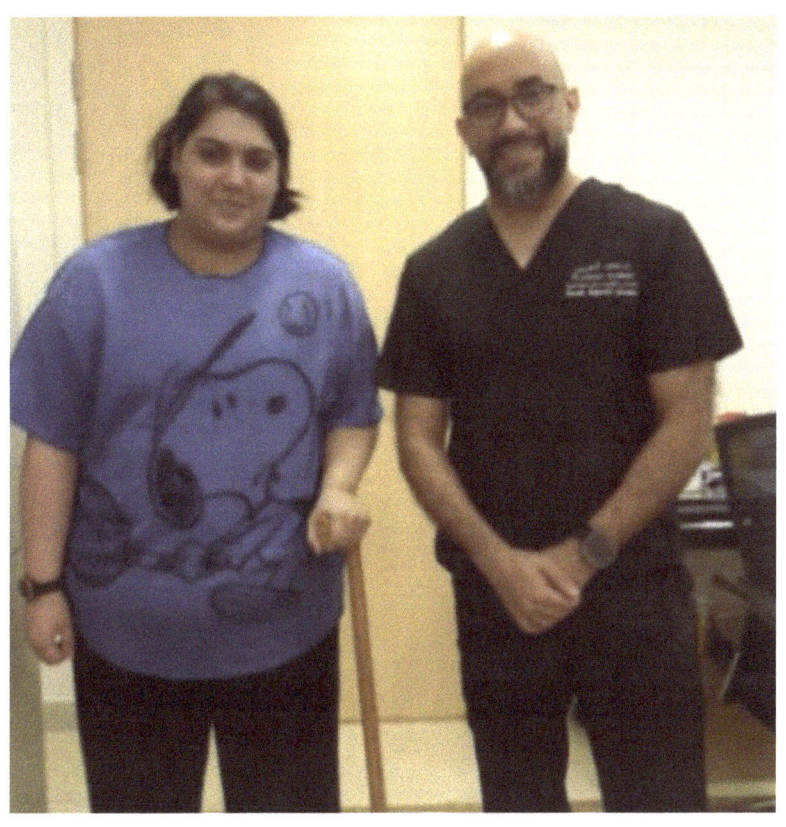

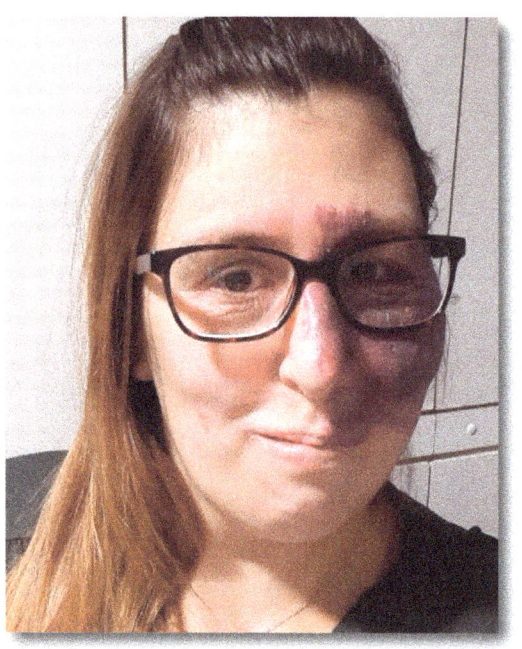

"Yes, I have a birthmark, and this has shaped my character, who I am, and how I think about certain things. Does that make me less or different from someone without a birthmark? NO. I am Penny, I hardly talk about my birthmark, I don't feel different, and I live my life as best I can."

# MY STORY, MY PAIN, AND MY GLORY

*Penny Pellens*

I was the firstborn child, and I arrived with a birthmark covering half of my face. Doctors told my parents at the time that this was from the delivery, and it would fade with time. Oh, how ignorant doctors can be. Doctors ask, "Oh, what happened to you? Wow, you really fell hard!" Nurses ask if they can help because I must be in pain. The ignorance of people who have studied medicine!!

I grew up in a family that did not discuss feelings, but that was probably normal at that time. Our parents didn't do this either, so why would they do it as a family? The topic of my birthmark was also taboo in the family. But I was the only girl on my father's side and had a wonderful grandmother and three aunts who spoiled me rotten. So I lived a normal childhood. Or, well, normal…

In elementary school, I woke up an hour earlier every day to cover my birthmark. I did this for almost my entire elementary-school years. When I see pictures of me from back then, I look like a doll wearing makeup and wonder how covering something actually made it stand out even more. Until I was ten, I did this every day, but then I had a moment when I asked myself, *Why am I doing this?* I then started a new life without makeup.

My high school years were like those of any teenager; I was searching for my own identity. Those were the years that teenagers can be cruel. The years when you develop a thick skin and try not to let it get to you. I spent two years at a boys' school and there developed a thick skin and a big mouth. I suffered nicknames like Gorbachev, got a bag of salt thrown on me because that "would get rid of the wine stain," etc.

Puberty was also the start of my first laser treatments. At a morning appointment to see what the options were, it was a bit of a push to have tests done in the afternoon. We just had to go for lunch and think about it. Which teenager doesn't want that big red spot gone from their face?? But I anticipated that it would hurt a lot, and I wasn't eager to undergo the tests. I remember getting glasses to protect my eyes, and after the tests, they were filled with tears from the pain. I found it inhumane pain, but the doctor said it would go away. So under pressure from the doctor, we started the treatment. The start of pain and misery…

Completely under anesthesia, two weeks not going to school, and especially a black, burnt face. I fell behind in school and had to repeat my year for barely any results. After one year and four treatments, I gave up and made peace with it.

The treatments also cost an immense amount of money. This was seen as a cosmetic procedure, and the health insurance didn't cover it fully. Thankfully, by 2025, they have made much progress in this area.

My puberty went by fairly smoothly. The big mouth was there, and so was the immense sarcastic shield. A circle of friends to go out with and always a boyfriend at hand. Later, when I think about it, I was quite popular, even though there was a different thought in my head at the time. Too little for someone, who would want me, look at my face…UNTIL I found someone in my friend group with whom I clicked, and he said the words that turned my whole life upside down. "Yes, you're nice and sweet, but your face…" That's when I decided that no one would be able to hurt me with comments about my face ever again.

A little later, I met the future father of my first two children. When the topic of children came up, I wanted to be sure it wasn't hereditary. I didn't want my children to experience a childhood like mine. It became a tumultuous relationship. Young, naïve, in love, and blind to the red flags. There was someone who cared for me, and I was someone who did everything to be liked. Needing to compensate. Always doing everything for everyone because that's how everyone would like me.

His narcissistic traits became more and more apparent, as did the alcohol problem. There were multiple instances of violence. Always on the side of my birthmark because that was already red/blue. So no one would notice. It was always my fault, according to him. After five years of terror, I finally had the courage to leave everything behind and start over from scratch.

After being single for half a year, out of sheer boredom, I decided to sign up on a dating site. Nowadays, there are plenty of apps, but back then it was quite a hassle through a website. *Oh boy, a photo and an intro. Shit, a photo… Everyone is going to see my face and judge.*

After some failed dates, I met a man I would marry. On my wedding day, my grandmother on my mother's side came in and said, "You haven't put on any makeup."

"No, I haven't done that for twenty years, so why would I do it for just this one day? Why should I hide who I really am? For nice photos of a person without a birthmark? My children would be shocked, and my partner has never seen me without it. So why would I do it?"

I still don't see the point in that. I don't want to offend anyone who covers up every day, but I don't want to present myself as someone I'm not. How terrible would it be to get to know someone and then take everything off in the evening and have them be shocked? No, thank you. The first impression is with the birthmark on my face. Take it or leave it. I understand that people do this, but I am who I am precisely because of that birthmark. Just like regular makeup or filters on apps nowadays. Why?? You are who you are. You are a person with character, and you are not defined by that filter or layer of makeup.

After nearly ten years of marriage, it ended when we were almost forty. The infamous midlife crisis. Another whole shit show of dating? No thanks! Which didn't even need to happen because one of my best friends became my current partner. When a friend suddenly died, I realized that life is way too short to be unhappy, and I chose to focus on myself to try to be happy and enjoy life. The divorce was finalized, a new relationship began, work was going well, and yet that midlife crisis was lurking around the corner.

The deep lows could sometimes feel like rock bottom. So I decided to work on myself and my self-confidence. Little by little, with therapy I realized that I could be who I was. That society has changed a lot and that talking about feelings is really okay. That you don't always have to bottle everything up, and when they ask if everything is okay, you don't have to automatically say yes.

I participated in a photo project about skin conditions and saw several little children with birthmarks. My heart broke every time I thought about how they still had to go through puberty. Hell is still waiting. I did several interviews for a newspaper and a lifestyle magazine about living with a birthmark. I was a big, tough person during the interviews, but when the publications came out, I crawled as far away as possible because I didn't want to read any reactions. Long live social media, where you can read everyone's unfiltered opinion everywhere. People really don't realize how hurtful they can be sometimes behind their keyboards.

But, thanks to social media, I have connected with others in similar situations from all over the world over the past years. I have seen tips, stories, and people, and I now realize that I am absolutely not alone. I also went back to a dermatologist, after thirty years, to have my face checked again. Over the years, I had developed bumps under my eye, my nose had grown crooked, my lip was very thick on that side, and my birthmark had indeed become very dark.

I was allowed to share my story about the past and what my current concerns were. Again, they wanted to do laser tests. My first reaction was no, absolutely not.

My boyfriend looked at me and asked, "Why not? You're here; the technology is also thirty years older."

So I decided to go ahead and do it anyway. The first little point catapulted me back thirty years, and my glasses were once again full of tears. The smell of burnt skin, the pain, horror… Until two weeks later…the result! Wow! Indeed, technology has not stood still, and the birthmark is much lighter where they tested. Only, now, I had a Windows logo test spot on my jaw. I found that worse than my birthmark

After the checkup, I decided to go for a full treatment. In my mind, I decided that I would have a maximum of three treatments. On our social security, I can have eight done without extra costs, but I knew I didn't want to take that long road all at once, so three was the magic number. In the meantime, I knew how I was going to look and wanted to spare my boyfriend and children from seeing that.

The first treatment went smoothly, although I still thought, *What have I gotten myself into?* as I was on my way home, wrapped up like a mummy. Suffering from a blackened jaw, applying ointment, taking painkillers, and resting—all quickly followed. Being as busy as I am, resting is not in my vocabulary. But everything for the greater good.

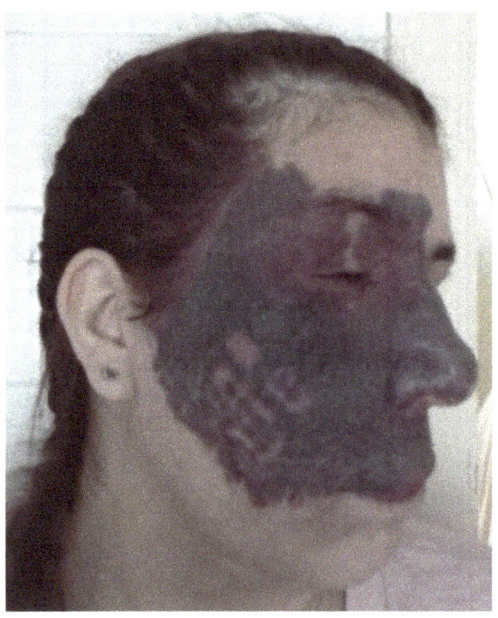

The second and third treatments were already scheduled. After the second treatment, I had a dip and decided to

cancel the third, or at least postpone it for a long time. Until I realized that if I postponed it, I knew it would still come... So I decided to postpone it for a month, and the third would be the last treatment.

Currently recovering from this last treatment, but already very satisfied with the previous two, I now realize how dark my birthmark had become over the years. For years, I proclaimed what a terrible thing that laser was; now, I would recommend it to people who are hesitant to do it. Does it change anything about me? No, because it is a part of who I am. Do people talk to me about it now? No, the subject is avoided. If I post before-and-after photos on social media, I get a heart or a "Wow, you can see the difference."

There is only a very small circle of three people who encourage me throughout this process: my boyfriend, my friend, and a colleague. They are there for me at every treatment and ask for updates in the morning, afternoon, and evening. My parents or family, you might be wondering? Well, they check in on how the surgery went, and maybe I hear from them the week after to see how I'm recovering. You know, avoiding the subject and not talking about the birthmark, feelings...

Did I consider getting lasered again in the hope that it would disappear? No, I buried that hope when I turned eighteen. It will never disappear, and I have truly made peace with that. Most days of the year, at least. Who hasn't had a bad day? Through people on Instagram, I see more individuals who look like me. Apparently, one in 300 is born with it. One in 300!! I'm not the freak they made me believe I was when I was younger. One in 300 people on this planet live with a birthmark! Even someone who passes by on my timeline makes me think, *Hey, I haven't posted anything. We look so much alike. Every indentation in our birthmark is almost the same.*

The group of people I have come to know is spread all over the world. People who are contributing to this book. People who understand what you are going through. You can tell your story, write it down, keep it to yourself, but these people know what it feels like to be stared at, to grow up with cover-up, laser therapy, all the discomforts… This is also true for people with freckles, red hair (my daughter has red hair, and I tell her all the time how beautiful she is!).

Every person has something they are not satisfied with. Sometimes it's visible, and sometimes it's not. I just happen to have the bad luck that it's on my face and immediately noticeable when you see me. Is a birthmark the end of the world? NO, absolutely not. Society is now completely different from thirty to forty years ago.

I don't see myself as less than or different from any other person on earth. Yes, I have a birthmark, and this has shaped my character, who I am, and how I think about certain things. Does that make me less or different from someone without a birthmark? NO. I am Penny, I hardly talk about my birthmark, I don't feel different, and I live my life as best I can. On good and bad days, I try to be charming and approachable. Sometimes, I overcompensate so that people, after being startled by my face, realize that I am kind and helpful. Sometimes, too much, because Doing Good for the Whole World is also my second name. I think I wouldn't have been this way if I had looked "normal." I often laugh and say what a Karen I would have been. But I'm glad I got this chance to show people that we are not different. We have a quirk of nature that stands out. There are many more people who have an inner quirk of nature that you only discover when you talk to them or live with them. With me, you immediately see what it is. Do people get startled? Yes. They stare, turn their heads, whisper; little children point; teenagers laugh, shout…

Can I handle it? Some days are better than others, but if they treat me with respect, I treat them with respect as well. If they ask questions, I will answer with my standard response: some people are born with freckles, and I was born with this, and no, it won't go away. Usually, kids are happy with this answer and go back to playing. While their parents stand by, full of shame. But why be ashamed? Childish curiosity and politeness are nothing to be ashamed of. Talking and showing emotions has taught me a lot, especially to be who I am and not hide away from anyone. Life is too short for that.

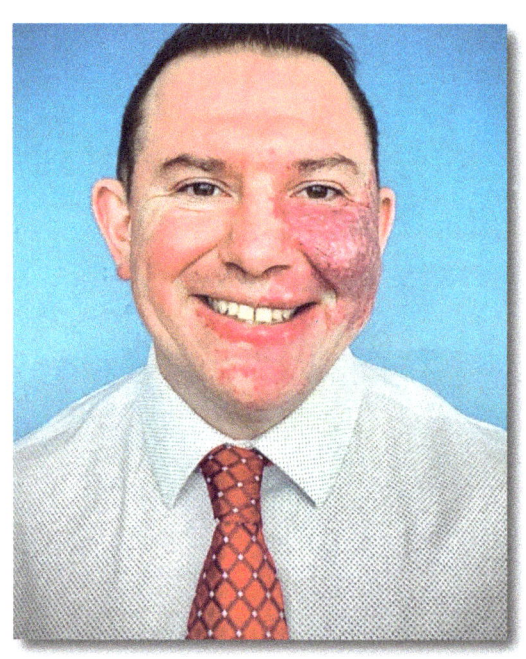

"Never let your skin differences stop you from accomplishing anything you want in life."

# HOW I FOUND YOU GUYS
## Dr. Scott Cupples

It was a warm October morning as I sat down on the front stoop to lace up my running shoes. At thirty-two years old, I was finding my rhythm again as an athlete, in hopes of putting myself in a better space both physically and mentally; 2016 was a rough year by all accounts, and I was focused on making a positive change in my life. I stood up and stretched quickly, activated my headphones, and started a playlist of energetic workout music for my three-mile morning run.

Usually, these runs are a great opportunity to detach from all the stressors in life and enjoy the beautiful weather. Even though the music was blasting, its intensity rising, my mind was silent except for one thing that kept rising to the forefront: for the first time in my life, I was going to have pulse-dye laser treatment on my port-wine-stain (PWS) birthmark.

A few months earlier, I faced a lot of adversity financially, professionally, and romantically and was in the middle of a deep rut. I was in the worst shape of my life physically, and probably mentally as well. After a real estate investment in which many lessons were learned, a rough breakup with my girlfriend, and a few hospital visits, I decided to start working out daily, which put me in a better space mentally.

One day, I had a random thought about my birthmark—how an old friend had told me there was a community out there that was prevalent online on social media platforms. I decided to search for it on Facebook and ended up requesting to join a group called It's Just a Birthmark: Port-Wine Stain Family and Friends. I was added immediately and continued my adventure as I scrolled through the various posts. I saw one post in which the mom of a young infant was emotionally asking for help and information about insurance. That reassured me. I also saw many adults with PWS posting everything from depressing cries for help to affirmations of pride in their facial differences.

As I continued my research, I discovered dozens of social media groups, from across the world, in which people connected through their shared experiences with vascular anomalies. Specifically, I connected most with those who had facial-skin differences like mine and saw that many shared the same experiences. I don't want to generalize trauma bonding, but in the military and in sports, I've noticed that going through adversity together forms the deepest connections.

PWS is a rare condition, and many who have a facial difference choose to cover it with makeup. Most people I encounter have never met someone who looked like me, which demonstrates how social media provided a platform for people affected by vascular anomalies to connect and develop a bond with people with shared experiences. Across the groups, friendships were discovered, and information was shared that provided not only medical treatment insight but social connections.

Personally, I always hated my PWS birthmark. When I was at my best, my mentality was that I was able to accomplish everything in my life despite this medical condition. I genuinely believe that the chip on my shoulder from having this condition has fueled most of the success in my life. As a child, I loved football and wanted to play quarterback. Well, the stereotype for that position is homecoming king (I will let you all paint your own picture of that image), and I was not the most popular, handsome boy in the school. Any lack of confidence from my facial difference was offset by sheer determination, which helped me achieve that goal.

As I moved through life and my career, I always looked at my PWS as something to overcome. At my lowest lows, I blamed my PWS for many things that I felt were out of my control. While I was often exceeding expectations in areas of life I could control, I still had to live with a large PWS on my face that resembles an injury more than anything. I never spoke about it publicly, and if asked, the most I would say about it is a brief explanation of how I have had it since birth. While I never covered it, it was embarrassing, especially when people loudly asked me what it was or made silly assumptions. At times, my PWS birthmark made me feel sorry for myself, and up until my social media searches, I didn't know there were people available who could relate.

The friend who told me about the birthmark community mentioned that my life experience would serve as a great example of an adult who has accomplished many feats, and it would be a good role model for everyone. That chip on my shoulder led me to some success in many areas, and I started to think about what I could do to make an impact. This made me think of my younger self and what a role model (who looked like me) would have meant to me while growing up.

I had never really given it much thought until that day that I joined the Facebook group. So on a whim, with minimal thought behind the message, I decided to post something in one of the groups:

> *We all have our low moments when dealing with our PWS birthmark...but you should never let your PWS hold you back from anything you want to achieve in life. Today, I reached a milestone by becoming Master Sergeant in the U.S. Air Force. Keep your head up brothers and sisters - use your PWS as motivation to fuel your success!*

After making the post, I thought little of it and went about my day at work in the office. Later that morning, I took a break and pulled out my phone for some mindless scrolling. To my surprise, I had hundreds of likes, many well-wishes, and a lot of inspirational feedback. I was taken aback by the response and started to scroll through some of the comments. There were so many congratulatory messages, introductions from people who were active in the group, and some who even expressed their appreciation for sharing my experiences.

The most profound message was from a mother of a child with a birthmark; she stated how important it is to have such role models in the community. She went on to explain how she showed her child (who has a PWS as well) my picture (in military uniform). The child's father was previously in the Army, and it seemed as if the child was ecstatic when she saw that someone like her could join the military and be like her daddy.

I was blown away by the response and decided to keep in touch with the community from that day on. I remember how I felt that day, which served as a pivotal moment in my journey of living with a vascular anomaly.

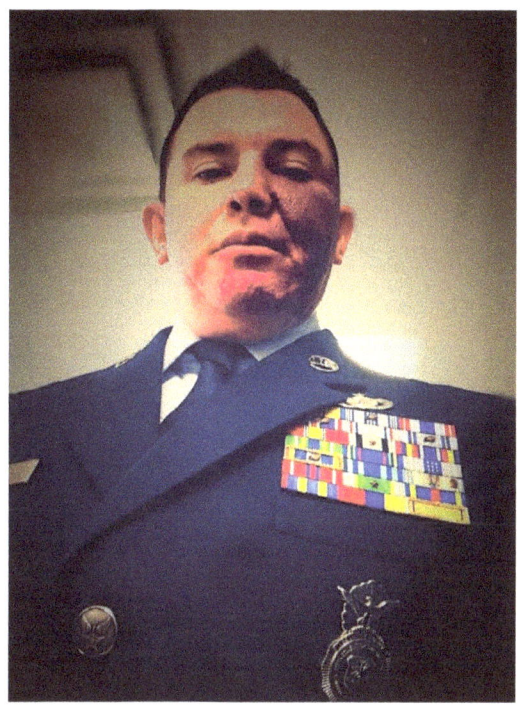

After I finished my run on that morning in October of 2016, I went inside the house to get ready for my trip to New York City. While I didn't frequent the city often, my nervousness was not about riding the train or finding my way around the big city. A nonprofit organization was hosting a conference, and they had coordinated with a medical office to provide free pulse-dye laser treatment for people with PWS. Months earlier, after talking it over with a few of my trusted friends I decided to register for the event to have my PWS treated.

As a child, you could see my freckles through my PWS, as it was very faint, smooth, and light. When I decided against getting laser treatment early in life, it was without the knowledge that my condition could worsen. A capillary malformation (the medical term for a PWS) is a progressive condition in which oversized blood vessels are present, making the skin look red.

They can lead to many health complications as they progress, which is what happened to me. Over the years, my PWS thickened, became darker, and grew nodules that even affected my peripheral vision.

As I studied my condition, I realized the gravity of not having it treated, so I decided to go out on a limb and register for the free laser session. I knew that one laser session wouldn't do anything, but at least it was a step in that direction. So here I was, thirty-two years old and taking a few days off work to hop on the train and get zapped in the face.

I sat there in the waiting room, numbing cream on my face, with a half dozen others. It was an awkward moment, as many of us were there for our first-ever treatment. I sat there in silence, waiting for my name to be called, for seemingly the longest sixty minutes of my life. Then Dr. Roy Geronemus and his team asked me some questions about my previous treatments, and I explained there were none. This turned out to be exciting for Dr. G, as I was a blank canvas for him to document his treatments on an adult who had received no previous care. He explained how he would cut and cauterize the nodules and then perform a laser treatment that would feel like rubber band snapping on my face. He went into detail about the effects of the laser, but at that point, most of the explanation went well over my head.

I don't remember much else about the treatment, as I tried to disconnect mentally to deal with the pain. It was over in a couple of minutes at most, which was surprisingly quick. The swelling and purpura from the laser stood out as I looked across the room into a mirror, but I also noticed that the nodules were gone. My first PWS treatment was complete.

That evening, I walked around the city and got some dinner by myself. While my face was extremely swollen, it wasn't as bad as the worst-case scenarios I had imagined. I kept to myself, wandering around the city until I discovered a Mexican restaurant for a nice dinner and a cold beer. I always get stares, but they felt more glaring that evening as I posted up at the bar table to enjoy my meal. My mind raced with thoughts about how I would explain the treatment to friends, family, and coworkers who saw me like this.

With that said, I knew it was the right thing to do. The nodules were gone, and I could see without obstruction from the growth on my face. After dinner, I started to take it all in as I walked around the city on that damp fall evening. Little did I know that the adventure had just begun.

The next morning, I walked into a lecture theater where, for the first time in my life, I saw more people in the audience with PWS than without. At that conference, I met so many people affected by various vascular anomalies and realized how important it was for people with shared experiences to connect. I spent hours talking to families, as they were very interested in my life experiences. I went on to share my accomplishments in the military, higher education, world travels, experiences with parenthood, and some general life experiences related to my condition.

Hearing these things did so much for the parents of those affected by vascular anomalies, as it gave them reassurance that their children could live a normal lifestyle. I knew at this time that I would have to find a way to make an impact on this community. Little did I know this would be the start of an amazing adventure in philanthropy, one geared around helping those with a vascular anomaly.

Almost ten years later, and fresh off a three-mile run, I found the inspiration to write this story for my good friend Hanna. I can genuinely say that I am proud to have found a niche in the vascular anomalies community, one from which I can help and support people and families affected. As a member of an amazing network, I've dedicated much of my life over the past ten years to the nonprofit sector that serves people with vascular anomalies and have supported events that provided treatment to people across the globe. My involvement with the vascular anomalies community's journey started with a social media post on January 19, 2016, and it continues with a recently created nonprofit organization, the Vascular Anomalies Alliance, for which I serve as chairman of the board.

My words to people affected by skin differences are the same as they were when I started. "Never let your skin differences stop you from accomplishing anything you want in life."

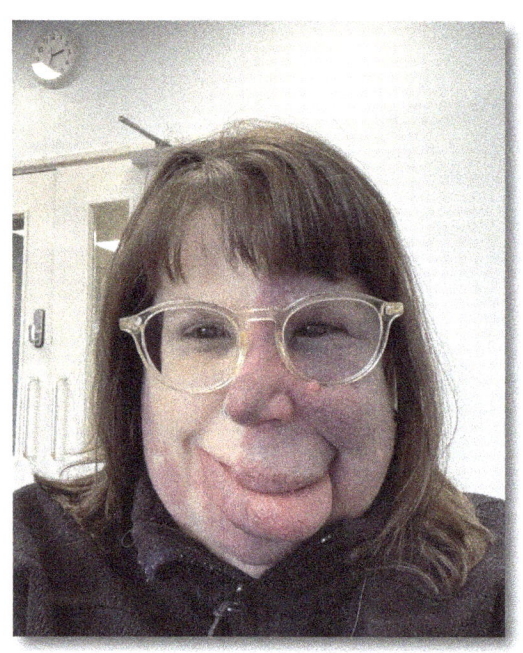

"I didn't know at the time, but the impact of looking after people changed me."

# MY STORY: FROM PATIENT TO HELPER

## Sharon James

You know those kids at school who had their life all planned out? The ones who knew what they wanted to do, and nothing was going to stop them? Well, I wasn't one of those kids. It's safe to say I had absolutely no idea what I wanted to do when I grew up. Maybe because I was a daydreamer, but mostly because, growing up with a large birthmark covering half my face and most of my body, I felt as if most jobs would be out of my reach.

I didn't have a lot of friends in elementary school. Some of the kids wouldn't come near me; they were afraid that they'd catch something, from being close to or touching my skin, and then they would end up looking like me. I had the odd bit of bullying, but thanks to a wonderful teacher, it was swiftly dealt with, and the bullies retreated to their caves and never bothered me again.

In high school, I was incredibly lucky that my older, popular brother was a year above me and in the cool crowd. If it weren't for him, I probably wouldn't be writing this; he was a great protector, and so were his friends. I wasn't in any crowd, not even the uncool one. I was just there, sticking out like a sore thumb, the only girl with a birthmark. I was lucky enough to make a few friends; decades later, they're all still in my life, and their friendships were and still are unconditional.

I digress. How did I go from clueless teenager to forty-something healthcare worker? It wasn't the most straightforward of career paths. I had a vague feeling about wanting to be a nurse. I actually applied and got into a nursing course after my high school exams. I was all set to start, but the college moved the venue to another location, several miles away. I was the stubborn, shy type at the time, and I decided I didn't want to travel outside of my comfort zone; it would have meant getting on a bus, one thing I avoided like the plague because it was guaranteed I'd be stared at by strangers. This was my sign that nursing was not for me.

I always had an interest in art and design as a kid, usually inventing horrifically corny brand names and drawing the packaging. I loved to draw; it was something I could do by myself, no one judging or commenting on my appearance. So I followed in my brother's footsteps and studied typographic design at my local college. I loved it. I still do. I felt as if I'd found my calling.

It wasn't until the end of the course that I realized how competitive the industry was. My confidence plummeted. It was the first time I realized that if your face doesn't fit, it doesn't matter how good your work is. Who in their right mind would employ someone who looked like me to present designs to clients? I've never had a competitive streak, and it was highly unlikely I would develop one overnight, if at all. I needed to work, but I knew I couldn't face applying for jobs in that industry.

I avoided anything that required facing customers. Supermarket? Nope. Receptionist? Nope. For a couple of years, I worked in kitchens of all kinds—schools, nursing homes, companies. It was easy money, and no one bothered me. In 1998, I hit the jackpot and joined the Royal Mail, the United Kingdom's postal service. I loved almost every minute of it. I had a uniform, which was made of the most uncomfortable, itchy fabric, but I didn't care. I felt as if I belonged somewhere; I was almost an equal.

Little did I know that my world was about to be turned upside down in 2009. My mum was diagnosed with breast cancer. It was a huge blow. The one thing that reassured me was how well she was looked after during her care. The nurses were incredible. As much as I loved my job and the people I worked with, I felt I needed a change. After thirteen years, I was offered voluntary redundancy. I took it and ran.

All those years I'd been afraid of being interviewed, and now my life depended on it. I applied to be a healthcare assistant, kind of like a nursing assistant, at my local hospital. There must have been something in the air that day because I got the job. Maybe it was my knowledge of the Ayliffe technique (handwashing) that ultimately won over the matron who interviewed me, maybe it was the way I completely faked my confidence—I'll never know. But the job was mine.

It was by far the best decision I'd ever made. I didn't know at the time, but the impact of looking after people changed me. As a child with a birthmark and a long-term health condition, I was regularly in the hospital. I hated being the patient; I felt vulnerable and scared. Now, I'm on the other side. I'm there caring for patients who are feeling the same way I did. It was as if I'd come full circle.

The thing with having a birthmark is that there are people out there who think it's their right to know, as they put it, "what's wrong with your face." Now, I don't mind people asking if they're polite and sincere, but when people catch me off guard, especially in the most inconvenient of places, such as while I'm doing my weekly food shopping, it does kind of annoy me. When people state, "Oh, that's a big red mark," depending on my mood, it will usually result in sarcasm or silence.

However, when I'm at work with a patient and they ask, it's like an icebreaker. It's something that I feel comfortable talking about because for a few moments, it might take away their fears and vulnerability. I will never forget one patient who looked at my face and promptly pointed at his stomach, proudly declaring his birthmark. It felt as if I were part of a secret club and meeting a new member.

Working in healthcare has changed me as a person. I'm no longer afraid of my own limitations or of shying away. I feel comfortable around my colleagues, and I feel respected, something I've never felt before. Knowing that I'm helping people who are going through the toughest times of their lives makes me feel as if I finally have a purpose.

Having a birthmark gives me a perspective that few others can see. It gives me a voice for patients who can't advocate for themselves or don't have the confidence to speak up because they're afraid or scared. It's a privilege that I never thought I'd have, and I can't imagine doing any other job.

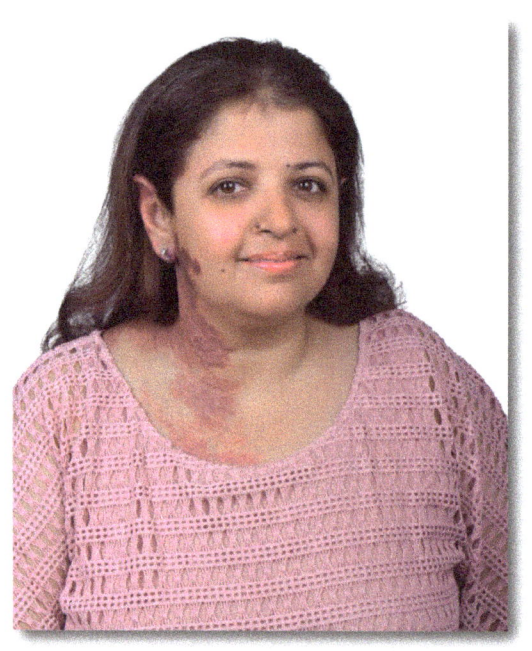

"As I write this, I realize I have to forgive my parents and doctors; that's the only way I can move on and eagerly run carefree to a life waiting for me."

# MY SIXTH SENSE: MY PORT-WINE STAIN

## Simran Kaur Dhatt

My mother tells me that when I was born, she was bewildered to see a big red patch on her firstborn baby's face, neck, and chest. It was a difficult pregnancy for her. I was born with the umbilical cord wrapped around my neck. The doctors had little hope that I would be born alive. I was a cesarean-section baby. My mother has never spoken about this. It was one of her childhood friends who mentioned this to me. My maternal grandmother, when she saw me for the first time, thought that I had been bitten by a mosquito on the face. She also had doubts that I had been handled properly by the nurses during birth.

Soon, the doctor put all doubts to rest and told my family that it was a birthmark known as port-wine stain. To give reassurance to my mother, the doctor suggested that as I grew up, my mom should get me a stylish haircut that would help to cover up my birthmark.

In India, your life is never private. Everyone is into each other's business. In my country, the concept of Mind Your Own

Business doesn't exist. Relatives and family friends came up with different theories and versions of why I had such a big birthmark on my body. The most common one was that it was very lucky for the newborn baby and the mother. The second one was that my mother had not been cautious enough during the solar eclipse and had exposed herself to the sun while she was carrying me, and this caused the big red mark.

Someone also said that an aunt had cast a spell on me. Oh wow! Now that I am writing it down, I feel like Snow White or Cinderella. Maybe even Alice in Wonderland. Alice falling down the rabbit hole. Alice living in her own world, away from reality. Though now I realize how important it is to live in the present and be aware of your environment, your surroundings.

I always felt different from my siblings and cousins. I never fit in. Now that I am a schoolteacher, I realize I have a learning disability. I was bad at mathematics and spelling. I always spelled *two* as *tow*, and *does* as *dose*. Once, a teacher thought it was very funny that I spelled *does* as *dose*; she mentioned it to the whole class, and my classmates thought it was funny too. It was evil of her, but that was a long time ago. I have never gotten myself tested for the learning disability. The last physical examination I had was in 2000. After that, nothing. I don't even want to.

In India, they also say that if you have been murdered in your previous life, in your next life you will be born with a birthmark on your body at the exact same place where you were attacked before dying. When I was a child, I dreamed of a newlywed woman in a red salwar kameez (traditional North Indian attire) and wearing a gold necklace, standing at the cobbler, waiting for her turn so that her shoes could be mended. This woman was with her husband and brother-in-law; they were supposed to go to a wedding together. In the last part of the dream, I remember the woman being scared of and being chased by migrant workers. And then the woman was strangled by someone. She was murdered for the gold she wore around her neck. That's all I can remember.

It's true; when something is said infinite times, it becomes a reality. I was always told by my mother and other family members that because of my birthmark, marrying me off would be a problem, a task. Well, that became my reality because the idea of trying to meet someone else's standards to appease them just didn't settle well in my system. To mold myself to be liked by another person—I could never do that. To survive, you have to be true to yourself.

Where I live in India, arranged marriages are about trying to make the prospective match and their family like you. Loving, caring for others, understanding others, and being patient have nothing to do with the way you look. Having been brought up in such a superficial social setting, sometimes I think I should have moved to another city or country to live a different life. It took me a long time to understand, deconstruct, and unlearn the idea of companionship. Maybe I am still learning.

I have memories about my birthmark from childhood. I remember going to spend my holidays with my aunt in Siliguri, West Bengal. I must have been seven or eight years old. On one occasion, I went to a dinner party with my aunt and uncle at their friend's place. During the dinner, I fell asleep. Someone picked me up and put me in the car when we were about to leave. Though I was half asleep, I have vivid memories of my cousin and another grown-up discussing my birthmark and saying how big and dark red it was.

When I was in sixth grade, a new girl came into our class. She had thick, short curly hair. We did not get a chance to speak to each other during the first few months of class. Then, one day, the teacher decided to assign everybody new desk partners. I did not want to sit near the new girl because she had curly, dense black hair. But eventually the class teacher made us sit together, and we became very good friends; we still are. She told me that when the teacher was changing the seating arrangement in the class, she did not want to be my desk partner because the big red mark on my face petrified her. I confessed to her that I was also wary about being her desk mate because I found her thick, curly hair rather strange.

When we come across people who are different from us, the human urge is to protect oneself from those physical differences or differences in opinion. Accepting differences takes effort, time, and an ability to adapt, learn, unlearn, and reconstruct preconceived notions. Throughout my teachers' training, we were taught "intelligence is the ability to accept and adapt to the changes in our environment."

I studied in a convent school from kindergarten through high school. When I was in second grade, a very affectionate nun named Sister Verona, on seeing my birthmark, asked me if I had been slapped by the teacher. I do not know on what impulse, but I ended up saying yes to Sister Verona's query.

During those years, there was so much terrorism in the region that I lived in. I remember, once, two armed men entered our school. There was no adult in our class, just around forty second graders. There was no noise in the classroom. No one spoke to each other for those two hours the men were there. It's very unusual for second graders to sit still for so long. I remember looking out of the classroom window, and I could not see any movement for the longest time. Eventually, I saw the school gardener coming out from the back of the building. I guess that gave me some sort of reassurance.

For the most part, school was uneventful. My classmates and the other students had seen me right from the beginning. They had long since accepted the way I looked. I did have some friends say strange things about my birthmark a few times, but I did not take them seriously.

In India, when I was in tenth grade, you had to sit for an exam conducted by the Central Board of Secondary Education. I was around fifteen years old then. After taking the exam, my parents decided to send me to England with my grandfather and younger sister. All three of us had our passports stamped for England, the United States, and Canada.

I remember sitting on the London tube and going for the doctor's appointment in Central London. We took a tube from Greenwich Village to, I think, somewhere in Central London. I was accompanied by my uncle, grandfather, and younger sister. The doctor looked at my birthmark and gave me an appointment for my first laser treatment in three weeks' time.

In those three weeks, we visited the USA and Canada. I remember my grandfather giving my sister and me a hundred dollars each to spend in the States. It was too much money for two kids back then; I think he did not realize that. I had a grand time spending all that money at the mall and Disneyland. My aunt on the East Coast also asked for my medical file so that she could show it to a doctor at Johns Hopkins Hospital.

We came back to London. The doctor at the clinic gave us an appointment. I recall my uncle purchasing a particular gel for me from Body Shop; the doctor had asked him to do this. My aunt drove us halfway to the clinic in her car. As there was a shortage of parking in Central London, she parked her car in a parking lot away from the clinic. We rode in a London Black Cab Taxi for the rest of the ride. It had white-lace curtains on the windows. It was so grand.

Sometimes I truly feel God made me Alice in Wonderland meandering through life. I was always a dreamer; my sister was not. She was rather practical, and that helped her reach her goals.

At the clinic, the doctor decided to do a test patch at the back of my ear. He also took blood samples and some other samples for examination. I remember the nurse holding my hand while the doctor gave me laser shots later that day. It was not painful; the doctor knew what he was doing. My aunt was also in the room; her presence was comforting and reassuring. My cousin in London was very concerned and anxious about my treatment, though she did not show it.

On the last appointment in London, the doctor told my uncle and me that it was best not to do any sort of laser on my port-wine stain. The laser available at that time had never been tried on South Asian skin. He also told us that the use of laser on South Asian and West Indian skin led to scarring. He suggested that I learn how to apply makeup. The doctor from Johns Hopkins Hospital (Maryland, USA) was also of the same opinion; laser had never been used on South Asian skin, so he did not want to risk it.

One day, five years later, my father heard on the news about a private clinic in New Delhi; they were using pulse-dye laser as a treatment for birthmarks. He got in touch with the clinic and booked an appointment for me. A private clinic should never have to advertise for itself in the news. Now that I look back, it was a red flag my parents missed. Maybe my parents did not know better; they didn't realize they should confirm the authenticity of this clinic and its treatments.

As I wrote about the pulse-dye laser treatments I received from 2000 to 2004, I started having flashbacks. It took me almost a day to get back to my normal self. I got nasty with my parents and ordered awful stale food from a local bakery. I told myself, *Stop complaining; be excited to meet yourself every day.* That helped to lift my spirits. I am at my workplace as I write this; a change of environment and being in the company of my colleagues helped.

Anyway, on the first day of the laser treatments at the clinic in New Delhi, my parents and I had very high hopes. My aunt in America sent a tube of the local anesthesia cream now and then, but after some time, she stopped, as it was causing problems with her health insurance. After about two years, her doctor in the States also told her that using so much anesthesia and undergoing laser every month would have consequences on my health and well-being. The doctor was definitely correct on that one.

On my first visit to the clinic, I was accompanied by my parents. As I sat there on the chair, I thought the treatments would be over after two or three sessions. Little did I know what I was in for. It was an unexplored journey, uncharted waters for my parents, the doctors, and me. I don't remember my younger sister in any way being involved in my journey. I guess sometimes siblings move away because they are too scared to be involved in your pain.

The first laser session was painful; the local anesthesia had been badly applied. I felt the laser on my neck. The doctor gave me so many shots at one time; if I remember correctly, it was around forty. I was in so much pain. I remember crying and the nurse holding my hand. My parents were there too. I have no idea what they were going through. The nurse told me to stop crying; she said that my tears might turn into steam if they came in contact with the laser.

Post-treatment care was so bad. My parents and I had no idea what to do. There was scarring…a lot of it. The doctor in

Delhi recommended a friend's clinic in my city as a place I could go for post-laser care.

For the entire four years of treatments, I don't even remember once having a decent cleaning of the wound. On the first cleaning, the doctor I went to used alcohol and tried to clean it. It was so painful I almost lost consciousness. I remember crying out in pain. I can't recall going for post-laser cleaning ever again. My wound was cleaned only on my next visit to the laser clinic.

Whenever I went out in the sun during summertime, I almost passed out. The sunrays were too strong. Excruciating pain and too many painkillers—I felt I was almost in a trance for those four years.

I dropped out of university for a year. Every month, I journeyed to the laser clinic with my parents. I found my original doctor to be very arrogant and eventually ended up having three doctors. The first one, the arrogant one, was in New Delhi. The second was a female doctor at a skin clinic in Ludhiana; she was arrogant too. The third one was in my hometown, Chandigarh. He judged me for not being focused on my academics and professional growth. That's the problem with a lot of Indian doctors; their degrees go to their head. Even if they are taught how to empathetically deal with their patients, the arrogance of having a doctor's degree overpowers the kindness in them.

Four years, a visit to the laser clinic every month—so if you do the math, that is forty-eight visits. Let's take out four visits. That makes it forty-four visits in four years to the laser clinic with badly administered anesthesia, ill-informed and inexperienced doctors, and my parents making me receive laser shots beyond my threshold, thinking it would speed up the process of making my port-wine stain disappear.

No, pulse-dye laser is not magic. From what I have seen and heard on the internet, it only lightens the birthmark and is used for maintenance. Please correct me if I am wrong.

The doctor in New Delhi stopped seeing me because I said mean things to him. His colleague in Ludhiana, a lady doctor, was my next doctor. I was her first port-wine patient; she had no clue about what she was doing. I remember she cleaned my wound with a fabric face towel after dipping it in water. I think that was very unprofessional of her. My parents did not like her. So when a branch of the same laser clinic opened in Chandigarh, my hometown, my parents started taking me there.

The rest of the laser treatments were done in the clinic in Chandigarh. Throughout the laser treatments, I just remember my ear and neck were constant wounds—pus, scarring, and at times oozing blood. That's what I went through for those four years. So much pain I couldn't function or accomplish the simplest daily tasks, my studies, or my job. Nobody understood me, not even my family. I was always judged for being behind in life. I did try therapy; that did not work for me. The therapist was too aggressive.

At the end of four years, I had to tell my parents the laser treatments must stop. It was an emotional and physical tool for my health. I was breaking down constantly in every human way possible. For the sake of my sanity, I had to make it stop. So I did. It took me the longest time to overcome the trauma.

As I write this, I realize I have to forgive my parents and doctors; that's the only way I can move on and eagerly run carefree to a life waiting for me. If I don't forgive, I will not be able to calm myself down enough to function well.

My friend, a therapist, suggested that I write about my experiences during those four years of laser treatments in order to help me overcome the trauma. I did just that, and I realized that the laser treatments are over, and in front of me lies a life in which I can do anything I want.

Recently, I went to visit an NGO for acid victims based in Noida. I told the victims that I felt as if no one understood me, not even my family. As the conversation advanced, one of the victims spoke about her post-burn experiences. The inability to come out of one's room and not even having the willpower to maintain basic hygiene. This resonated with me.

The manager of the NGO said to me that she felt I was looking for people who had similar experiences as mine. She was definitely right. The people at the NGO suggested that I visit a café named Sheroes, which is operated by acid-attack victims in Noida. At the café, I met the manager, and we had quite a conversation. He told me his perspective of my laser treatments. In his view, my parents had tried to do their best for me. They tried as hard as they could to do whatever they thought they could do to give me a better life. He also said that I had held on to the trauma for too long. It was time to let go.

Yes, twenty years later, it is time to let go. To take responsibility for my feelings and emotions. No one else can do it for me. To try my best to fall in love with myself. To be excited to meet myself every day. To look forward to each day and what it brings to me.

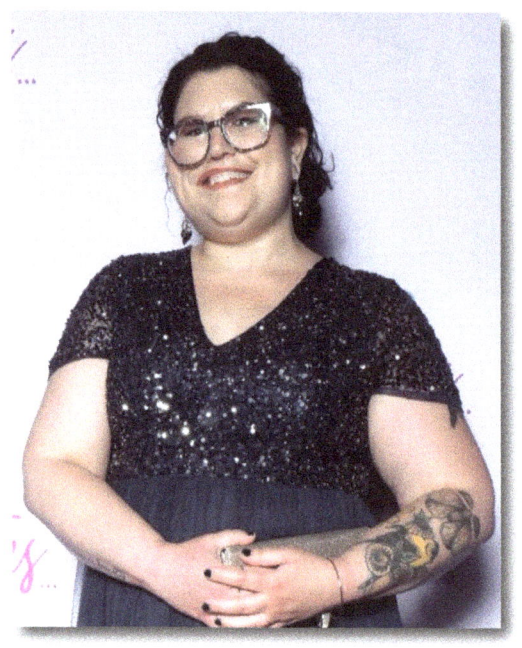

"The mask comes off. It's time to just accept that this is you, this is the way you look, and you look beautiful."

# SMILE AND SAY CHEESE!
## *Tiffany Kerchner*

Say that to most people, and they'll follow your command with no questions asked. We smile and take pictures when we're happy, right? We take photographs at weddings, birthday parties, bar mitzvahs, and the like. We want to capture the moments of joy and happiness. We want visual memories to look at with a loved one and share that moment in time and the joy we felt.

Photographs, videos, cameras. Things I wanted to hide from as a child. Although I have photographs, I have many memories of happy and joyous times in my life. That's until someone gets the camera out. Why? In a world of Mona Lisa smiles, I am a Pablo Picasso.

This is how I went from a rough draft to a masterpiece.

This next statement I am about to make is one I've made hundreds of times.

> *Hi, my name is Tiffany. I'm a typical millennial American and live in the rural Southeast Pennsylvania. I'm a nurse by day and a bookworm by night. I was born, on a Friday, with a rare neurological disorder called Moebius* syndrome.

*If you've never heard of my condition, I'm not surprised. Two out of every one million people will develop this condition. It's me. Hi, I'm one of the two; it's me. In short, Moebius syndrome is the absence or underdevelopment of the sixth and the seventh cranial nerves, which results in facial paralysis. This condition affects the right side of my face. This condition took me down a rough journey. This condition led to many photographs of me. It led to people painting my face.*

When I received this diagnosis as a toddler, my mother went on her own journey of putting a name to what was happening to her baby. Many doctors' offices, specialist after specialist, and never resolving the issue. Until I landed in the hands of Scott Bartlett, MD, a plastic, reconstructive, and oral surgeon and the director of the craniofacial program at Children's Hospital of Philadelphia.

He informed my mom that due to the structure of my face, over time the paralysis would eventually result in my skin drooping. They kept saying that I couldn't smile, which I never understood because I knew I smiled. I knew I smiled when I was at dance class. I smiled when someone hugged me. Why were they saying I couldn't smile? Still, my surgeon and mom stood there and talked about making me a smile. He explained that there were a series of reconstructive plastic surgeries that would start at age six. My mom went ahead with the surgical options.

If you've ever had any kind of reconstructive or plastic surgery, you know the drill. You go into the office; your surgeon comes in and talks about how to fix what is broken. They stand there talking about your biggest shame and insecurity. They take many pictures to log the process. *Snap*. Every flash of the camera is a reminder that this is happening because you're damaged goods; you need to be fixed. You can't even smile. The morning of every surgery, your surgeon and artist draws all over your body, indicating where they need to make incisions, what goes where, etc. You are the subject. They put on the anesthesia mask; you start at ninety-nine and count down. *Snap.*

Even though I had this condition, I was still very much a child, a human. I still had needs and wants. I still deserved to be loved and treated with respect. I went to grade school like every other child. Although I was bullied a lot in school, I liked school. I liked learning, and I loved having friends. My favorite subject was always English and literature. I also enjoyed music and art classes. It was hard being the kid at school with a facial difference, but everyone got to know me, and it seemed a lot of people accepted me. I didn't have to explain my existence.

Enter picture day. The day I always dreaded. I didn't mind putting on a dress or having my hair done. It was the awkward experience of having a new person enter your school. *They don't know about me. Are they going to stare and call me names too?* So waiting in line for pictures, the anticipation builds.

It's finally my turn, so I sit down on the stool in front of the backdrop. The photographer takes one look at me and gives me what I call "the look," the "oh, this is curious" look, the one that reveals shock, sometimes fear, sometimes disgust. He says, "Smile," so I smile. Then he says, "Give me a real smile," thinking you're one of those prankster kids who is making a silly face just to be defiant. But I am smiling. This is my "real smile," so I say sorry. I apologize for existing. I just want to get this over with. He finally snaps the photo, and it's over.

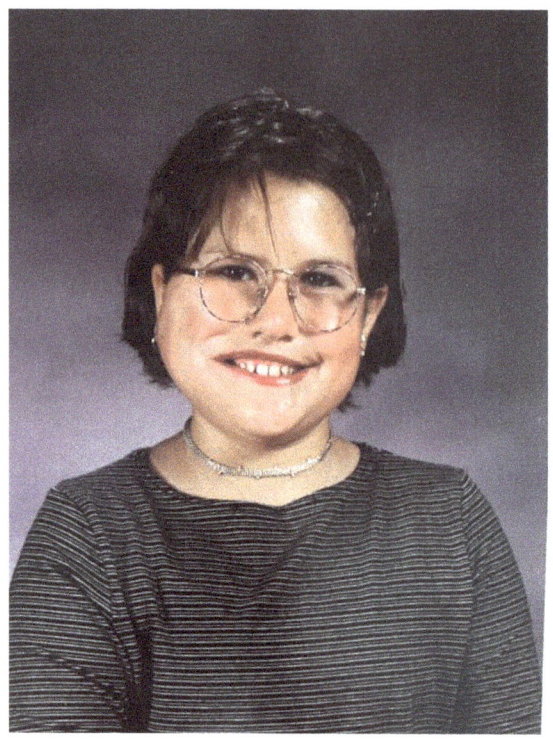

I was enrolled in dance lessons as a child; I took tap, jazz, and ballet. Every summer, we'd have an annual recital as well as perform for groups and other venues. The big summer recital, you get to get fitted for costumes. You get your hair and makeup done. *Snap.* You feel so beautiful in your shiny new costume. They take professional photos. So much for being happy and excited. You get the pictures back, and everyone in your class photo looks so beautiful. Except you. You stick out; you're different; you need to be fixed.

Today is your birthday, a day every child is excited about. You get cake and get to open presents. Then it's Christmas, the second-best day of a child's year. Everyone is taking pictures. *Snap.* You're reminded of how much you hate having your picture taken, but you smile anyway. After all, you did just get the new Spice Girls Barbies and soap and lotion from

Bath and Body Works—cucumber melon, of course. The family photographs aren't terrible. My family knows me. They know what my smile looks like. They accept me. Birthdays and holidays are good. *Snap.*

But then you get invited to a friend's birthday party. A new set of people. A new set of faces staring at you and asking you, "What's wrong with your face?" Because my face is my greatest shame. It's "wrong"; it must "be fixed." But it's your friend's party, and there are other people there. You hear them whispering about you. Then your friend's mom wants to take pictures, and all the moms want to take pictures. Smile; say cheese. *Snap.*

But you don't want other people taking your picture. You don't want their friends and families asking about you. You don't want to give anyone more of a reason to talk about you. You're a little girl. You have manners; you're polite. You smile and have fun. Then you go home and crawl into your bed and cry. Because no one can see you cry.

School. Parties. *Snap.*

Dance recitals. School dances. *Snap.*

Then you finally reach your senior year of high school. It's a tradition to have professional shots taken. You bring a few different outfits. You get your hair and makeup done. *Snap.* They show you the shots. Then they show the beauty of Photoshop in 2007. They photoshop your face to make it look "normal." There was no preparing me for this. It was just "Look at how beautiful you are," but also "Look how I can make your greatest shame go away." You say to them, "But that's not my face; that's not how I look. Please don't do that."

Enter social media. A place where not only your friends and family, but also complete strangers all over the world, can judge you. But you don't worry because by now you're eighteen. You have tricks up your sleeves. You turn your head so your difference isn't as noticeable. You wear your long hair down to cover your face. If you zoom in close, your difference isn't as noticeable. And that's the face you show the world. You don't feel safe showing your real face. Smile. Say cheese. *Snap*. Life goes on.

You use social media to stay connected with your friends and family all over the country. You're not one of those influencers. They're in shape. They're beautiful. They're not you. *Snap.* You start seeing women with facial differences too. You're in awe of their beauty. You stare at their pictures. You wish you could be beautiful like them. *Snap.*

Then, one day, a spark—not a snap—occurs. You see a woman with a facial difference; she's talking about having a facial difference. You're intrigued. You're inspired. Because by now you're in your thirties, and you still have a hard time talking about it. Because talking about it would mean acknowledging it. And you live in a fantasy world where you look like everyone else.

But something about the women in social media brings out a new side of you. You are so inspired. You look at yourself in the mirror and say, "If those women are beautiful, and they have a facial difference, then that means you are beautiful too."

The mask comes off. It's time to just accept that this is you, this is the way you look, and you look beautiful. You, too, start talking about your differences online. Making videos mostly for fun. You share your heart with the world. You find people, and people find you. You make so many connections. Every time you have an interaction with another person with a facial difference, it's this instant connection. "I see you. I feel your pain. I know." It is truly one of the most magical experiences. It feeds your soul until the work is complete, and you're reminded that your face is a masterpiece.

So you're not Mona Lisa. But you are you. People come from all over the world to gaze upon her, to find the meaning behind her infamous smile. One of the greatest mysteries. What is it that she is thinking? I like to think she, too, found her own beauty; she became her own work of art.

*Snap.* Smile. Say cheese.

# ABOUT THE AUTHORS

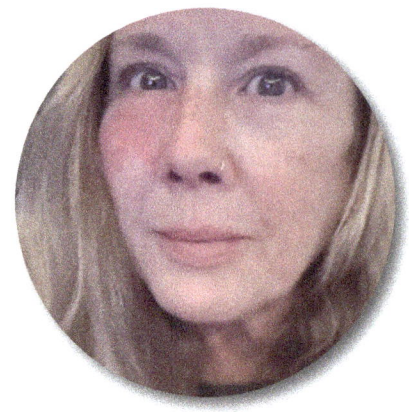

**Ana Lankford** is a born-and-bred Okie who has spent the majority of her life on red dirt. She is the mother of three, two sons and one daughter, and is the 'amma of one perfect little granddaughter. Ana also has a three-legged, blind pug she adores and two not-that-smart cats. Ana works in the substance-abuse recovery sector as the executive director of a private high school and recovery support program, working with teens and their families as they navigate the journey to sobriety. She loves her family, the beach, and sunshine.

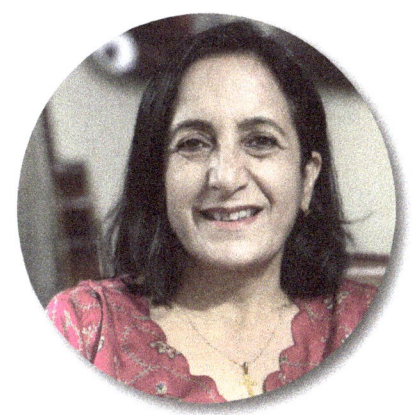

I am **Batool Kaushal** from Bhopal, India. I was born with Klippel-Trenaunay syndrome in Kashmir. KTS is the rarest of rare disease conditions. Having gone through so much in the last sixty-one years, I continue to be optimistic about my future health.

I have an MPhil in the philosophy of language and a teaching degree, and I worked in the public sector until I was diagnosed with breast cancer in 2020. I am also a trained pranic healer. I am the mother of a twenty-five-year-old daughter, Tanya, who is a journalist in London. My husband is Indian Army Veteran Brigadier R. K. Kaushal.

My hobbies include swimming, golf, gardening, and cooking. My happy-go-lucky attitude keeps me going.

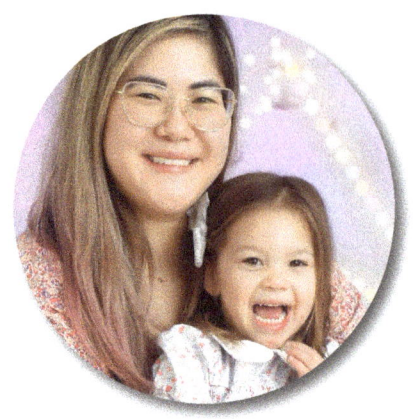

**Crystal Gordon** is a busy mom, wife, and jill-of-all-trades. She graduated with honors from the University of New Mexico with a BA in journalism and mass media communication and an MA in elementary education. She is actively involved with a couple of communities she feels passionately about. Crystal promotes positive social change and spreads awareness for the vascular-birthmark community. She also uses her voice to speak out against the abuses occurring in the unregulated troubled-teen industry. In her spare time, she enjoys traveling with her family and trying new restaurants.

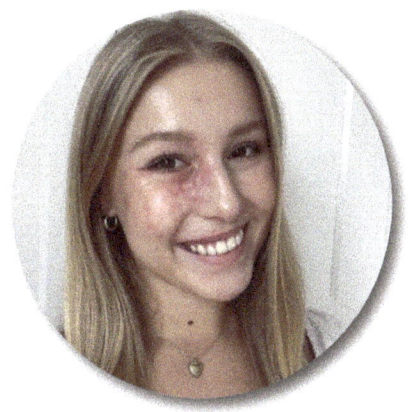

**Dana Marie Rückert** is a nineteen-year-old from Frankfurt, Germany. She is in her final year of high school and plans to pursue a German state law degree. As vice chairwoman of her local youth council, she actively represents young people's interests, advocating for meaningful change in her city. Her passion for understanding systems of governance and justice naturally aligns with her commitment to advocacy. Living with a port-wine stain, she shares the perspective of a young person embracing self-acceptance and confidence. Through her writing, she hopes to inspire others to embrace their differences and challenge societal beauty standards. Beyond her advocacy and studies, she enjoys playing soccer and tennis, going to the gym with friends, and exploring new perspectives through travel and reading. Follow her journey on Instagram: @danarueckert.

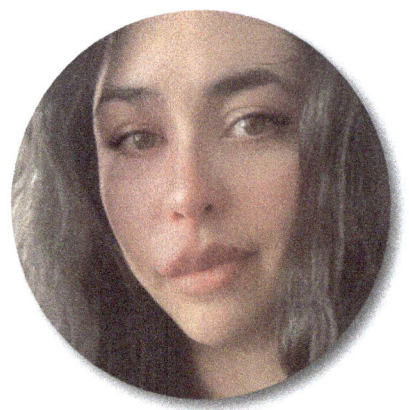

**Hanna Prangner** was born in McAllen, Texas, and moved to El Paso, Texas, with her family when she was two years old. She studied at Western Tech to become a medical biller and coder. Hanna is a mother of two daughters and enjoys being close to her family. Hanna has a passion for writing and loves being involved in the birthmark community. She enjoys connecting with the community and being able to learn as well as continue to spread awareness.

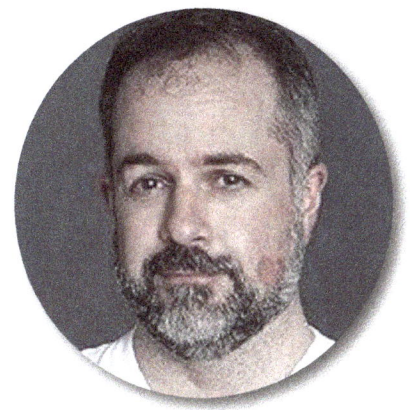

**J. Brian** is an actor/writer/jack-of-entirely-too-many-trades. A people person who admittedly finds people dubious, he is best described as "It's complicated." He lives with his wife, three dogs, two cats…and is worried there's a damn squirrel in the attic.

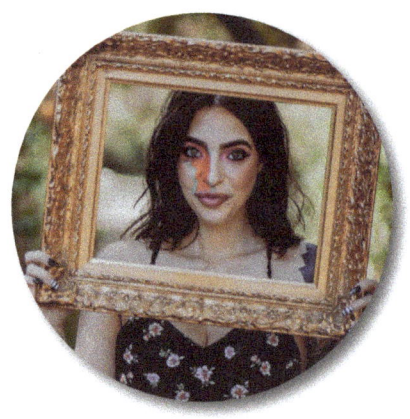

**Jessica Weckherlin** is a passionate light worker, entrepreneur, and advocate dedicated to helping others embrace their inner power. As the owner and beauty alchemist at Badass Beauty and Healing, she blends her expertise in beauty and wellness to create transformative experiences. She also cofounded the Badass Soul Collective, a soul-aligned business in which she and her best friend empower women through digital courses and healing retreats. A certified transformative breathwork facilitator and intuitive healer, Jessica guides others on deep journeys of self-discovery and healing. Her work extends beyond business; she is a global ambassador for the Vascular Birthmarks Foundation, advocating for awareness and support. Most importantly, Jessica's greatest work is being a mother to her daughter, Adelaide. Whether through beauty, breathwork, or sisterhood, Jessica is devoted to uplifting and inspiring those around her.

You can follow her on Instagram:
@badassbeautyandhealing

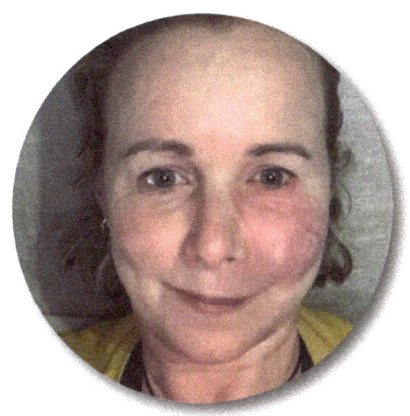

I am Kirsty Heather Ferguson, a primary school teacher, and have two daughters, Ally and Zoë, and a partner, Josh. They are my forever cheerleaders. They encourage me to be me. When we were going through tough times, we had a motto we used together—Be Brave, Be Bold, Be Brilliant, and Be Beautiful. I am so lucky to have them on my team. My family—Zoë, Tweeds, Griffy (aunt and uncle from Ozzie), Josh and me, Mum, my brother, Josh (Ally's partner), Ally, and my dad. Ally and Zoë have always just seen me as me, unperturbed by how I look or the color of my skin. They have never listened to the "bad side of my face" analogy. My partner, Josh, has always just loved me for me. My face and port-wine stain are irrelevant. He has allowed and encouraged me to be my authentic self, and I am grateful for that. He makes me feel content.

I did want to be an artist or laser surgeon but wasn't guided in those directions by my teachers. So I decided to become a teacher to ensure that I helped kids realize their talents and encouraged them to go for their goals in any way possible. I am an excellent teacher and have a superpower for bringing out the best in kids. I am also a big supporter of those kids who are different, be it quirky, ADHD, or neurodiverse. I worked in my own business for ten years, tutoring teachers and students with dyslexia and dyscalculia, and I loved showing them how clever they were! Ironically, I have recently been diagnosed with ADHD and am starting meds. This has helped calm my inner voice, which made me believe in myself. For the first time in my life, I am able to accept a compliment instead of downplaying it.

I enjoy surfing (a newer hobby), traveling either in New Zealand, Australia, and Southeast Asia. I LOVE saunas, walks, and painting/making T-shirts. One day, art will claim a bigger piece of my life; for now, it is emerging more often, and the ADHD meds have helped the creative brain have the juice to focus, explore, and create.

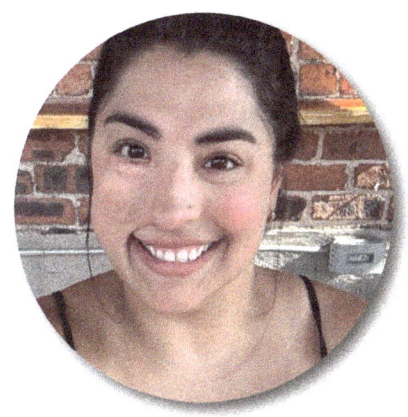

**Lorena Bryant Hixson** is a former ER nurse turned entrepreneur and mindset coach dedicated to helping women break free from overthinking and self-doubt. After struggling with confidence due to a visible scar, she embarked on a journey of self-acceptance, learning to embrace her story instead of hiding from it. Now, she empowers others to step into their worth, set boundaries, and build lives that feel authentic and fulfilling. As the founder of ShelfCare Box and Undoing the Nice Girl, Lorena shares practical tools and no-BS mindset shifts to help women stop people-pleasing and start prioritizing themselves. When she's not working, you'll find her exploring New York City, lost in a book, or blasting Taylor Swift.

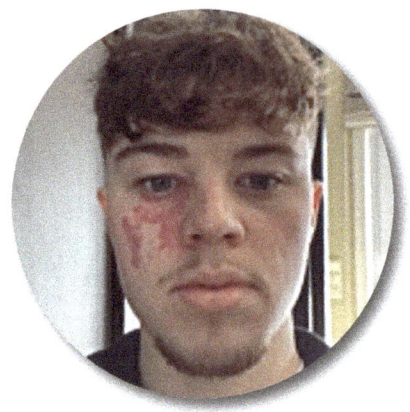

I'm **Matthias De Potter**, the founder of Aspilon, a medical-grade cosmetics brand designed for people with skin conditions. Born with a port-wine stain, I spent years searching for makeup that truly worked—something quick to apply that offered a perfect skin match, was long-lasting even through an active lifestyle, and was good for my skin. But nothing met all these needs. Most products were cakey, short-lasting, or even made my skin worse. After testing countless options for over a decade, I decided to create my own. My mission is to develop breathable high-performance cosmetics that don't just conceal but care and give people confidence without compromise. Because I know firsthand what it's like to need something better. And now, I'm creating it.

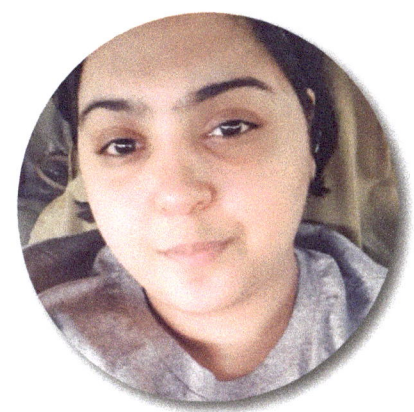

Hi, my name is **Omaima Aladwani**, but just call me Om. I am from Kuwait City, and I am twenty-eight years old. Here are some fun facts about me: I love traveling, meeting people from different cultures, and learning languages and history. My first language is Arabic, and my second language is English. I understand the Turkish language, but I don't speak it well; I will learn it soon. I love reading, going to the theater, editing, drawing, and listening to music.

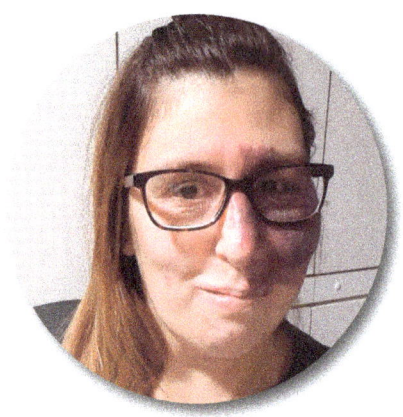

Hi, I'm **Penny Pellens,** born in 1981 in Belgium with a birthmark on the right side of my face. I have one son, two daughters, and three stepdaughters, so quite a bunch! As an office worker for a waste management company, I live between numbers and can really indulge myself. I've always had a fondness for numbers and practical solutions to keep life running smoothly. In the little free time I have, I enjoy planning weekend trips, coloring mandalas to relax, reading books, and spending time by the sea with my partner, whether it's for a walk or a bike ride. The ordinary family life that we love. I don't like being in the spotlight, and I enjoy the peace and quiet in our mixed chaos that prevails at home.

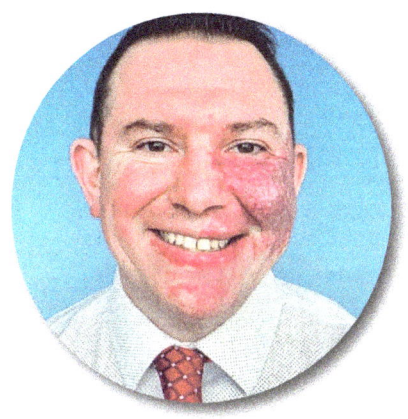

**Dr. Scott Cupples (DBA)** is a student and practitioner of organizational leadership. He gears his life around increasing the scope of his impact on helping others through his dedication to the organizations he serves. Mr. Cupples has served twenty-two plus years in the military, achieving the rank of Chief Master Sergeant in the United States Air Force National Guard, with 400 plus airmen under his charge. Scott has recently cofounded the Vascular Anomalies Alliance, a nonprofit organization supporting the vascular birthmark community through education, treatment, and community support. He is an avid traveler with a thirst for adventure and dedicates most of his time to parenting his son, Dohnovan, as a single father, serving his country, and supporting his vascular anomaly community.

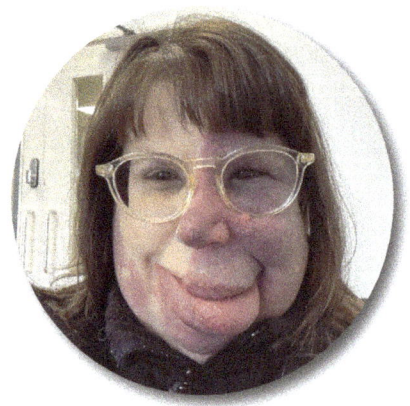

**Sharon James** is from England, United Kingdom. She is based in North London and works as a physiotherapy assistant for the National Health Service.

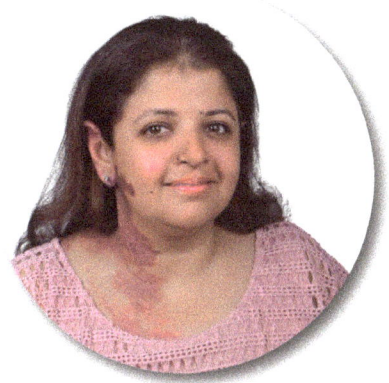

**Simran Kaur Dhatt** has a port-wine stain on the right side of her face, neck, and upper back. Simran lives in Chandigarh, North India. She is forty-six years old, has a PhD in education, and is a kindergarten teacher who enjoys gardening, cooking, trekking, and reading.

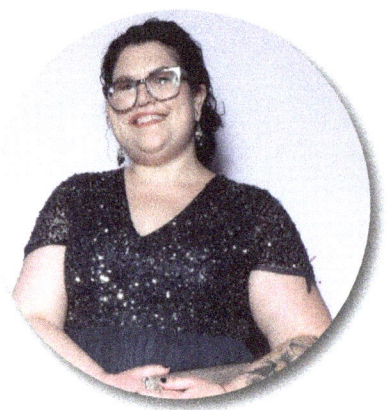

**Tiffany Kerchner** is a thirty-five-year-old from Philadelphia, Pennsylvania. She was born with Moebius syndrome affecting the right side of her face. She is a nurse by day and a facial-difference advocate on social media by night. She hopes to empower people with facial differences to love and accept themselves. You can find her either reading a book or gardening.

www.ingramcontent.com/pod-product-compliance
Lightning Source LLC
Chambersburg PA
CBHW040300190426
43198CB00050B/2940